The Immune System, Autoimmune Diseases & Inflammatory Conditions

Improve Immunity, Eating Disorders & Eating for Health

Anthea Peries

Copyright © All Rights Reserved.

Version 1.1 – March 2022

Published by Anthea Peries

ISBN -13: 978-1987794687

Disclaimer

This document is geared towards providing exact and reliable information in regards to the topic and issue covered. The publication is sold with the idea that the publisher is not required to render an accounting, officially permitted, or otherwise, qualified services. If advice is necessary, legal or professional, a practised individual in the profession should be ordered.

From a Declaration of Principles which was accepted and approved equally by a Committee of the American Bar Association and a Committee of Publishers and Associations.

the information is without a contract or any guarantee assurance.

Any trademarks that are used are without any consent, and the publication of the trademark is without permission or backing by the trademark owner. Any trademarks and brands within this book are for clarifying purposes only and are the owned by the owners themselves, not affiliated with this document.

Table of Contents

About this Book

You know how you seem to catch colds several times in a year? Alternatively, perhaps you continuously feel run down, listless and tired. Maybe, you have an upset stomach or an addiction to certain foods, perhaps pains in your joints. There could be reasons for this.

If you want to know how the immune system functions, what are autoimmune disorders and conditions, and how you can maintain a healthier body, then this book is for you.

There are ways to improve your immunity against inflammatory Conditions and even eating disorders. Health is more than looking fit; the right weight, shape or, following yet another crazy, fad diet. We are what we eat, and it is most important to find out exactly how the immune system works.

Yes, genetics and environment can play an active role in your lifestyle, but what we eat is essential too.

Our immune system gets taken for granted and yet; it does a lot for us, its primary function is to protect us from illness, viruses or diseases. If we do not look after our immune system, we can become sick. Our immune system needs our support too so that it can function properly.

This book will explain the immune system functions; how it becomes impaired, what are autoimmune diseases, what is proper nutrition, types of deficiencies and toxins to avoid, tips on eating healthy, how you can improve and strengthen your immune system, alongside other benefits.

Before you embark on any form of immunity improvement or diet plan with the help of a medical professional, it is crucial to understand basic immunology.

The immune system is an incredibly vast network of cells, tissues, and organs that coordinate your body's defences against threats to your health. Without a healthy immune system, there is no protection against billions of bacteria, viruses, and toxins that would transform anything minor from a paper cut or a seasonal cold, fatal.

So how does the immune system work?

The Immune System

The Immune System

The ancient Greek scientist called Archimedes considered the amount of water in the proportion of his body while he sat in his bathwater and this later evolved into the principle of the immune system.

Scientists researched how our cells communicate that there's an infection in the body. How does the body know where to send an aspirin for pain relief such as a headache?

Communication is carried out by eight vital sugars, not the table sugar type either. These eight sugars are significant for proper immune system functions.

All cells have molecular structures called antigens which are like ID tags. Each ID tag informs the immune system if a cell or other structure is good or bad.

A simplistic explanation might assist here.

Immune system cells move throughout the body stirring other body cells and asking the cells questions:

- *Do you belong to this body?*
- *Are you keeping well?*
- *Do you require any help?*

It is the sugars that the cells use, to code the conditional response answers, so that the immune system can understand the cell's answers. Through this sugar code; eight glyconutrients, the cells answer either Yes or No. If the answer is No, to the first question, the immune system presents an attack upon the foreigner, which is an immune system rebuff of the unknown intruder.

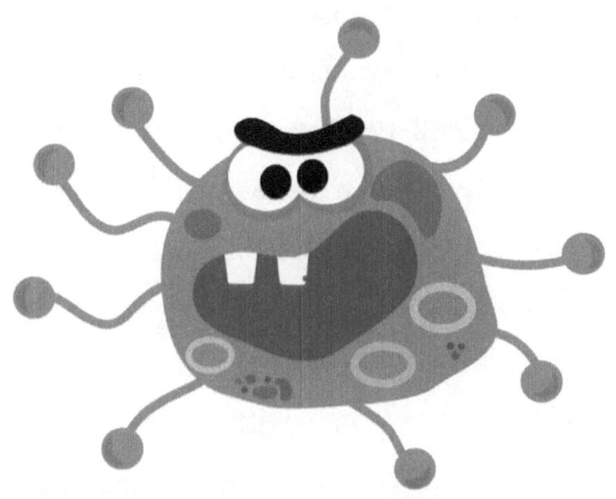

Unfortunately, intruders or foreign bodies can mutate, so the immune system receives a signal that is unusual, and it must then wait for more developments. Mutation is the reason we have different types of colds and flu, discussed later in this book. Such events involving immune system cell response might increase or speed up with a pre-prepared supply of glyconutrients.

If the cell responds with a "no" to the second question, i.e., are you keeping well? The immune system then sends for help, repair, or protection.

Should the cell answer "no" to the third question, i.e., do you require help? The immune system cell will move on to further cells.

Healthy cells that contain the eight sugars send out the right signals for the path of nutrients, i.e., elimination of toxins. The removal works with the immune system, assigning antibody assistance; requirements for dismissal of dying cells within the immune system; signals of abnormal growth from the immune system.

Alternatively, should the immune system not function properly (sugars are not present or prepared nutritionally or are malformed), we have one of several immune system responses:

Overactive Immune System

Here is an example of the immune system is an *overactive* immune system, we might develop allergies:

- Asthma
- *Diabetes*
- *Eczema*
- *MS*
- *Lupus*
- *Psoriasis*
- *Rheumatoid Arthritis*

Under Active Immune System

Without sugars present, we may have an *underactive* immune system condition. An underactive immune system issue could develop into:

- *Bacterial or viral infections*
- *Bronchitis*
- *Cancer*
- *Candida (yeast)*
- *Colds*
- *Ear infections*
- *Flu*
- *Hepatitis B and C*
- *Herpes simplex I and II*
- *HIV*
- *Strep*
- *Sinus problems*
- *TB*
- *Urinary and other infections*

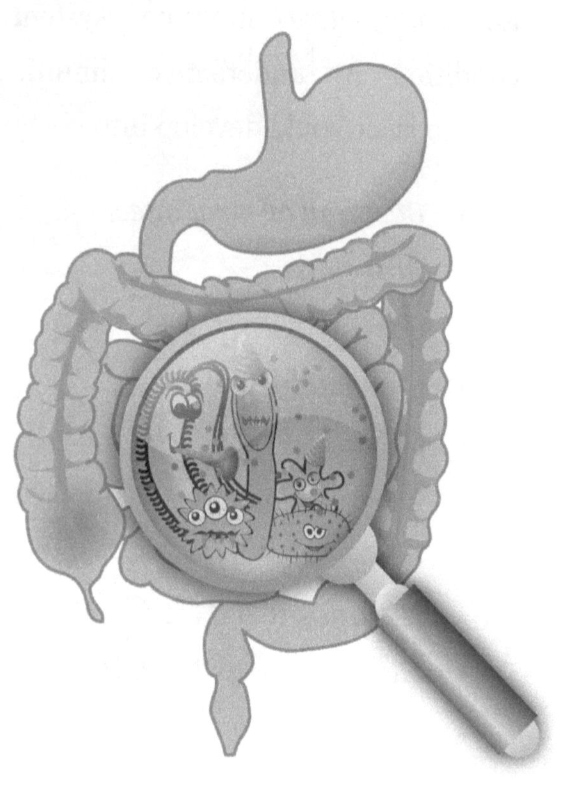

So you see, glyconutrients act like modulators for our immune system. Therefore, should the immune system get overactive, these modulators assist in *adjusting* and *balancing* the immune system reaction. Alternatively, the immune system has an underactive immune system; the glyconutrients present in the system are then able to boost the immune system's power and strength.

Providing the body with glyconutrients can mean significant help for the body's immune system when dealing with viral, bacterial and fungus infections; malignancies, parasites, and neurological issues.

Lastly, glyconutrients considerably increase immune system killer cell reaction by at least 50 percent in some people, who are usually healthier; this means decreasing infections, growths, and parasites. Statistics have shown that people with compromised immune systems are as much as 400 percent more likely to pick up germs.

Immune System & How to Support it

- *Do you understand what your immune system does?*

- *Do you know the parts that make up your immune system?*

- *How does it all work?*

Those are the things that we will now explore and more.

What is the Immune System

The immune system protects the body; it is a complex defence mechanism system. A pathogen; virus or bacteria that enter the body; the immune system finds, kills and removes the pathogen. The immune system prevents the body from disease developing.

The immune system is a multifaceted system of complex interactions concerning numerous organs and glands in the body, also substances like lymphatic vessels, bone marrow, white blood cells, and serum factors in the blood. Our immune system relies on all of these components to function cooperatively.

How your Immune System Works

The immune system separated into two areas:

1.   *The innate system*
2.   *The adaptive system*

Innate Immune System

The innate part protects you from infection, and it is continuously present and acts as the first line of defence.

The innate immune system includes dendritic cells, macrophages, and neutrophils. There are Natural Killer

Cells (NKC's), involved in the innate immune system. These destroy cells infected with a virus; this includes cancer cells.

Moreover, the innate immune system comprises skin mucous membranes, also other parts, to defend health by blocking out and inhibiting pathogens.

Adaptive Immune System

The adaptive immune system is the side of the system that adjusts and adapts to respond to anything that might pose a threat to your health. This area of your immune system is the reason why you may not get the same standard cold virus more than once; this includes chickenpox.

The adaptive immune system has two fundamental mechanisms:

- *antibodies*
- *T-cells*

These identify exact types of bacteria, virus-infected cells, and other pathogens.

Please be aware that there are many outlines on how the immune system works.

For an accurate and detailed definition, refer to a medical site, encyclopedia or medical book.

Nutrition & Your Immune System

There are many kinds of nutrients which are necessary for the function of our immune function.

Here are just a few of them:

1. *Glyconutrients are a significant part of the immune reaction. Glyconutrients get used to form glycoproteins, which shield the outsides of all cells in your body. The immune system uses these glycoproteins, besides others, for identifying pathogens.*

2. *Phytonutrients fight disease too. Scientists are not yet entirely sure about phytonutrients used by our body but have a direct effect on a condition, or both.*

3. *Colostrum used as a supplement has been known to help boost the immune system.*

Deficiencies in Vitamin C Can often cause poor Immunity too. Hopefully, you will at least have a slightly better basic understanding of the immune system, and how it functions.

You can see why it is essential to make a significant effort to support your immune system with a proper diet and natural supplements.

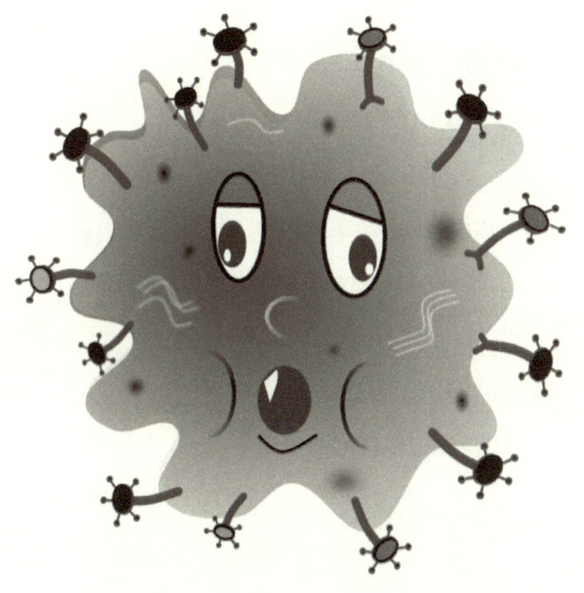

The Immune System Needs Support Too

The human body is a fragile and vulnerable organism, aside from the line of defence which the immune system provides to protect it as much as possible. Without a natural defence mechanism, the bacteria, microbes, parasites, toxins, viruses, etc., would diminish, and compromise the body to its chemical components in a short time.

The immune system works twenty-four hours all day every day; it never stops unless you are dead, and it never seems to get a spotlight on the work it does; taken for granted almost. However, should the immune system fail us in some way, we sure notice it though.

Environment (Nurture)

In our environment, we seem to inhale and eat many thousands of germs each day, while our immune system stops them from triggering diseases. However, when a virus sometimes breaks in through the immune system, we can end up with an illness. After the immune system familiarises itself and learns about these germs, it can fight them off, and we get over the condition.

The main parts of the immune
system:

- *bone marrow*
- *complement system*
- *hormones*
- *lymph system*
- *spleen*
- *thymus*
- *white blood cells*

The immune support system exhibits
dual characteristics:

- *self or non-self recognition*
- *general or specific*
- *natural or adaptive*
- *cell-mediated or humoral*
- *active or passive,*
- *primary or secondary*

Certain parts of the immune system can fight against specific antigens. These particular parts are known as *antigen-specific.*

Additional elements of the immune system are systemic, that is working through the human body instead of restricting themselves to the initial infection area; while others identify antigens to attack when they become a threat again. Such parts of the immune system are reported to hold some memory.

Genetics (Nature)

All of us are born with a natural defence system that is genetically based. The skin is a significant organ of our natural defence system. Any wound is like a doorway for germs to come into the body. The incidence of a foreign object inside the body enables the immune system to take action; eliminating the invaders while the skin eases the wound. If this process does not happen, the outcome result is an infection.

Bites and Stings

Another indication of the immune system functioning is when for example we get swelling or a rash on the skin, after mosquito bites or bee stings. There is no doubt the body would eventually come to a halt without the immune system.

Here are some of the things that could go wrong with a sub-optimal immune system:

The self or non-self recognition mentioned earlier in the immune system happens when every cell shows an indicator founded on the major histocompatibility complex (MHC). If a cell does not show this kind of marker, then the immune system treats it as a non-self and therefore, attacks it.

Attacking its cells

An analysis of this process and its results, causes the immune system to attack self-cells. Multiple sclerosis, systemic lupus, certain types of diabetes and arthritis are all *autoimmune diseases* caused by the immune system attacking its cells.

Allergies can be the result of the immune system exaggerating and overeating to particular stimuli.

Diabetes

Diabetes occurs when our immune system attacks the cells in the pancreas and terminates them. Also, rheumatoid arthritis is the result of the immune system affecting the joints. The immune system can cause problems during organ transplants; it can often refuse consent and accept the new organ.

Encouraging the immune system to be in good working order, especially with the ever-increasing levels of toxic pollutants in the environment, is quite a tough task.

Recent research has led scientists to think that particular carbohydrates signify the next cutting-edge solution in their search for non-toxic compounds that help to maintain the immune system.

The eight of essential sugars, called glyconutrients, already discovered and only two out of these can be found in our daily diet plan, however. These eight essential sugars provide the body with glycoforms needed for cell-to-cell communication. In medicine, the last four out of eight Nobel Prizes awarded for research into Glycobiology.

A constant amount of glyconutrients is required to keep the immune system functioning well. The body seems to recover and heal much quicker with glyconutrients if administering, for example, chemotherapy and radiation.

These same environmental toxins that weaken our immune system additionally affect the body's capacity to blend these glyconutrients; the reason why we need to ensure a constant supply of these glyconutrients via glyconutritionals or food supplements, which contain glyconutrients.

Our living conditions have become increasingly polluted in this world. The body is undoubtedly finding it had to fight off the bad-effects of this through its natural processes. So it seems that it is down to us to find out more about advance medical information to help our body to cope better.

How Do Probiotics Strengthen the Immune System?

Probiotics are bacteria or yeast that is good for you, especially for your digestive system. Certain bacteria are healthy for you. Your body naturally carries the right types of bacteria.

Probiotics are called "good" bacteria because of their significant alignments for your digestive system or gut. There is about a kilogram of bacteria in our intestines which have about over 300 different species. A few of these bacteria are the "good" ones. These bacteria are always fighting against each other, and when the dangerous and harmful bacteria outnumber the good ones,

this is when you can experience
digestive issues.

Some of these problems may include:

- *bloating*
- *chronic constipation*
- *tiredness*

Probiotics have an essential role to play in regulating proper digestion and intestinal functions by balancing the group of bacteria and microorganisms known as microflora.

Keeping the Digestive Organs Functioning Properly

Around 70% of immunities found in the gut region. Your gut is one of the open portals to the internals of your body. The disease usually begins internally; you can catch a cold; you get the flu, etc. As a significant open portal, other infection and conditions can also creep inside' with food and drink too. So it makes sense 70% of the immunities; your 1st line of defence, in your body found in the colon.

How do probiotics help us?

The thing that aggravates your colon is bugs.

Negative bacteria

Over time, if left unchecked, harmful flora becomes an overwhelming force in your body. Probiotics will affect the harmful bacteria in the colon, but the overall parasitic load in your body is now in overload mode, i.e., no amount of probiotics will reverse the trend; it only treats the problem in the gut or colon.

Therefore, you must manage the whole parasitic load in your body; otherwise this parasitic load will feed off the area in the colon, and this makes the probiotics virtually useless or using probiotics only treats the colon, and therefore only provides temporary relief.

So, probiotics strengthen the immune system by keeping the cells of the colon clean. Which means immune system; cells in the colon are not under attack from parasites or bugs. This condition allows the immunities and the cells of the colon to work as they stay healthy and are not laboured or under attack from an invader, foreign substance or parasites.

Unfortunately, the overall floral content of the body must be appropriate and not overloaded with harmful flora. If this is the case, then the bad flora in you; feeding the colonic area and probiotics are just a patch or band-aid.

If you restore the floral content of your body so the bad flora cannot gang up and pick on the colonic area, then probiotics are more efficient than we know, have experienced or been taught by the health industry. Maybe they want you to take their drugs, their products and spend money needlessly.

If you get your overall floral health balance right, you would not believe how much less you have to take their medications, if you take your probiotics and keep your gut health right.

What to Search for in Probiotics?

What you need to know about probiotics

It appears that how you look and feel might be directly related to your intestines. Encouraging better health in this area requires your intestinal tracts to take in nutrients adequately, and help eliminate waste and also toxic substances.

Your intestinal tracts, which lie between the belly as well as the rectum, are part of the Gl tract or digestive system. In the smaller as well as large intestines, food is broken down and taken it into the bloodstream, giving your cells and organs the energy to function.

Your intestinal tracts do this with the help of good germs (likewise called microflora).

These "great microorganisms" aid digestion, promote significant nutrient production, preserve pH (acid-base) balance, and stop the expansion of unwanted bacteria. From birth, your body becomes inhabited by less harmful bacteria. Modifications in your diet regimen, undergoing stress, and anxiety, as well as ageing and other variables, can disrupt this subtle, delicate equilibrium.

The absence of suitable microorganisms could result in:

- *Digestion issues*
- *Poor bowel function as well as unwanted gas*
- *A deteriorated immune system*
- *Poor vitamins and mineral absorption*
- *Low level of power and health*

The absence of significant germs is so usual that many wellness specialists recommend the use of probiotic supplements. Probiotics are good germs that restrict the expansion of unwanted bacteria in the digestive system by crowding them out.

In the very first years of the twentieth century a Russian researcher, Elie Metchnikoff, recommended that the long lives of Bulgarian peasants may be a result of their consumption or incited bacteria which affected the microflora of the colon. This exploration, together with he operates in immunology, made him the 1908 Nobel Reward for Medicine. This event increased considerable interest in the research study of advantages of bacteria to human beings.

In 1974 the term "Probiotic" (pro meaning for; bio meaning life) was coined to explain the use of helpful bacteria to influence health as well.

Today the clinical field concurs that probiotics offer a broad series of wellness advantages when absorbed in adequate numbers.

Restoring the balance

We may have few of these microorganisms in our gastrointestinal system, which in fact is usual but when it occurs, our bodies let us know with signs like occasional slowness, abnormality, bloating, or a weak body immune system.

There is a synergistic partnership between good germs and our body:

- *we provide them with a safe place to live and expand*

- *they aid us to digest*

- *absorb our food*

- *eliminate and preserve a healthy intestinal function*

Strain Uniqueness

However, not all probiotic germs are identical. They vary by type, varieties, stress and also results. Additionally, microorganisms should both live and colonise within the gut to induce significant effects. Sadly, many probiotics do not even reach the intestine and hence provide no benefits at all.

Practicality

Probiotics are breakable live germs. Probiotic cultures differ, and the advantage of a probiotic is not determined merely by the number of living microorganisms in a pill. The advantageous effects of the existence of probiotics in the gastrointestinal system depend upon their stability-- the ability of the bacteria to make it through, as well as conquer.

In the U.S. several probiotic products supported by enough research study, are poorly developed, as well as experience low-quality control. Many items list bacterial genera and varieties but not refer to the viability of the germs. Acidophilus, for example, has about -A 53% viability, which means that only half of the bacteria you take will have the ability to endure or last.

So, you need to consider whether it is worth buying expensive probiotic supplements if they are not useful.

Strengthen the Immune System Naturally

As we already know a properly functioning immune system is vital to our health. It is central to the healing process, whether it be a small scratch, a multifaceted virus or disease; the ageing process interlinked with the immune system too.

A weakened immunity leaves anyone open and vulnerable to diseases, and this then impairs our ability to heal in the right way and to age well in good health.

Signs of impaired immune function:

- *Allergies*
- *Candidiasis or yeast infections*
- *Chronic diarrhoea*
- *Chronic fatigue*
- *Inflammation*
- *Recurring infections*
- *Listlessness*
- *Slow wound healing*

Those who have suffered from up to three colds or infectious illnesses in a year most likely have a weakened immunity system.

How does our immunity become impaired?

Regrettably, modern living contains things that can weaken and damage our immune systems such as:

- *Chemicals in household cleaning detergents and sprays*
- *Chemotherapy*
- *Environmental pollutants*
- *Food additives*
- *Poor living conditions*
- *Pesticides*
- *Overuse of antibiotics*
- *On-going stress*
- *Poor nutrition*

Several disorders linked to a compromised or weakened immune function, such as:

- *Diabetes*
- *Lupus*
- *Pernicious anaemia*
- *Thyroid deficiency*
- *Heart disease*
- *Rheumatoid arthritis*

For peak immune function we first need to identify any disorders that might be hindering the immune function. Also, we should take precautions to circumvent any exposure to toxins like chemicals and pesticides that we may use in and around the home.

You can wear gloves perhaps while cleaning, to avoid exposure to the skins, and limit inhaling fumes from cleaning sprays, bleach, and the like by wearing a mini mask around your nose and mouth when cleaning.

Ensure the glassware and dishes get thoroughly rinsed out from any residual dishwashing liquids and so on. Although expensive, you might think about buying non-toxic detergents and cleansers. Try to take small steps like these whenever you can and try to ensure your shampoos and soaps made from natural ingredients where possible. Lastly, it is essential to have plenty of fresh air

and to drink plenty of the purest
water you can find.

Your Body Wants to Fight the Flu

Our body immune system is the initial line of defence against any attacks from bacteria, germs, and viruses such as flu. The immune system identifies any harmful invaders in the body and starts the process of first isolating and then destroying them one by one. However, the immune system will only work if it has the right fuel that it needs to function correctly.

As we already know, the immune system is known as a system because it comprises numerous organs and sub-systems that labour together in complete harmony.

To recap again, the primary parts of the immune system include:

- *Antibodies*
- *Bone marrow*
- *Complement system which is about 30 specific proteins that circulate in the blood plasma*
- *Hormones*
- *Lymph system*
- *Spleen*
- *Thymus*
- *White blood cells*

Every single part of the immune system is dependent on proper nutrition so that it can work at top efficiency. So should one component of the immune system under-perform, the rest of the entire system might be at risk of dysfunction.

An immune system that fails will leave the body with no protection from attack. It is the reason why AIDS and HIV are such devastating diseases.

Some diets that do not provide the minimum of nutritional levels that the immune system needs to do its work might be the main reasons why when the next flu season hits it might be the next worst. Individuals from developed countries, for example, have diets that are too high in saturated fats and too much sugar; low in vitamins and minerals. Many underdeveloped nations suffer from malnutrition and starvation. What is certain is that most individual's immune systems are not even prepared to combat the latest flu threat.

You do not have to allow your immune system to fail you. You have options, and instead, you can provide your body's immune system with exactly what it needs to function at peak performance, and you can do it without a particular diet plan by having to eat a range of unique foods or ingesting handfuls of vitamins and minerals.

Prepare and winterise your body by eating the right foods more regularly or by taking just one multivitamin capsule per day. Make sure you first chat with a doctor or a qualified herbalist before you take any supplements.

☐

Dangers of Influenza

There is one particular danger awaiting its victims in winter, and often that is flu or influenza. This horrible illness is known all over the world and in the USA, people do not appear to know much about it, especially and the cause or consequences of having this virus. We will discuss more on this issue.

Flu is transmittable, and most school children are aware of it. It is the most widely spread disease especially in the countries with a moderate climate. The initial symptoms are fever, cough and running nose. The sheer exhaustion of the condition and continuous state of tiredness or sleep is usually the first sign that a person may have become infected. You might think it possible to ignore the symptoms, allowing your body to recover naturally, not so, this is the type of disease that, if left untreated can cause severe complications, and in the long run, could be dangerous. The many difficulties are pneumonia and tuberculosis. These diseases are very contagious and perilous. There seems to be no other prevention as an alternative except for vaccination. If you need to be vaccinated, there are many things you could consider. Protection needs to be carried out about three months before the possibility of an outbreak of flu. It takes time for the cells to work out the immunity against this disease.

There are other ways to decrease the risk of getting infected. You need to be living a healthy life, getting rid of bad habits. They can destroy your immune system and make you extremely vulnerable to catching flu.

Fortunately, natural methods can protect you too. Garlic, for example, is a mighty powerful in fighting against diseases. Not many people are willing to eat it except in the form of seasoning perhaps but, it is tremendously useful in boosting your immune system, against several significant infections. You can also find syrups by companies which contain herbs that can encourage your immune system to become stronger.

However, be mindful and be aware of public places, if possible because these are the place you can instantly pick up germs. Carry alcohol soaked wipes or jell with you at all times, to disinfect your hands and any objects you use.

Some people have to be vaccinated, and it is compulsory; this can assist in preventing the spread of the disease especially the vulnerable.

These people are usually over 55 or in some countries over 60-65, as they are considered to be a member of a senior community. Those for example who had an operation on their thyroid, as I had several years ago, in some cases the immune system is much weaker and needs assistance to fight off the disease.

Another vulnerable group might consist of small children under the age of 7. They seem to be in close contact with others, and besides, their body is weak and unable to boost their immune system. The prevention of influenza is a significant issue these days, and there are new government programs around to help improve medical treatment.

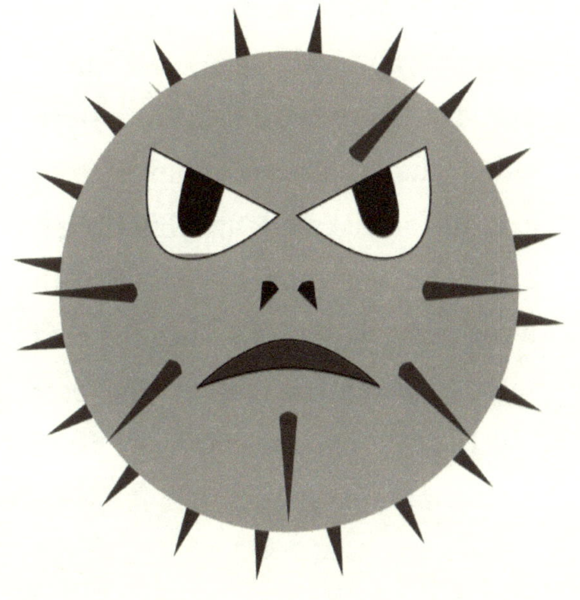

Colds and Flu Against a Robust Immune System

It is an achy, awful feeling having the flu when every single muscle and bone in your body aches and hurts. You cannot get a good night's sleep either, and you have no appetite to eat, and it takes a long while to get better, but you cannot be in bed with it for a few days only. Once the cold season descends upon us, the best way to protect your self is by having a robust immune system.

We know our immune system acts as a shield to protect our body from the bacteria, germs, and viruses that can bring about the illness. So, if our immune system is weak, the more vulnerable we become to getting sick. The stronger our immune system, the better we protect ourselves from getting ill. It does not mean that we will not catch a cold, but with a stronger immune order, we will undoubtedly be far better able to fight off any illnesses much faster.

So, how will we build up our robust immune system? What we can do to make our immune system healthy and vigorous.

I have mentioned before, the first is nutrition, and we all heard of the saying, "garbage in, garbage out" when using a computer for example?

The same applies to our bodies. Terrible eating patterns will result in limited diet, which won't give our bodies the right vitamins, minerals, and nutrients that it much gets to stay healthy and active. Now and again a good old cheeseburger or ice cream is okay, but of course in moderation which is the key.

Regrettably, the best nutritional habits do get defied to give the body with what it needs; to build a robust immune system.

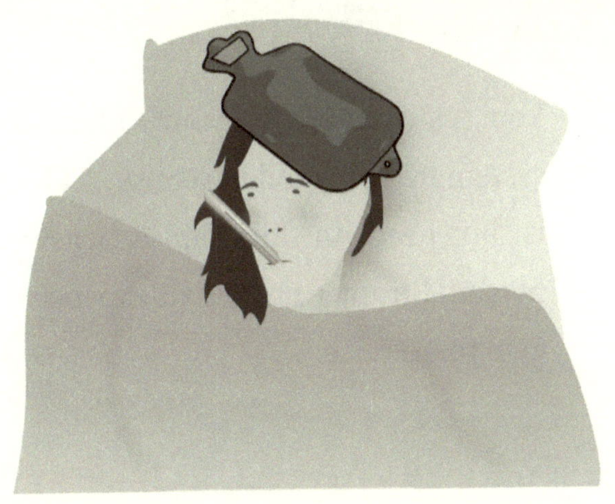

Nutritional supplements, like vitamins, minerals, and immune system boosters can help where even proper nutrition cannot.

Exercise

You can improve your immune system by doing mild exercise. There is no need to hire an expensive personal trainer or join an expensive gym to exercise.

Do you notice how invigorated you can feel after a pleasant long walk? Regular walks, bike rides; swimming, gardening, and of course yes housework are all wonderful ways to exercise.

However, there are things to avoid as we know, like excessive smoking and stress that can weaken and compromise the immune system. People who often experience high-stress levels in a work environment, for example, can feel awful and get sick more easily and often.

Building a healthy immune system does not happen overnight. It has to be something that we continue to develop and maintain our entire lives. Therefore, we will be far less prone to getting ill.

To be able to fend off illness and lead a better quality of life, in the long term, start today and build your immune system towards maintaining good health.

Other Steps to Improve Immunity

Good Nutrition

Besides using herbs to build up, balance and strengthen the immune system, it is vital to supply the body with enough nutrients:

- *Vitamin C is essential to the body's defence system otherwise known as the infection-fighting vitamin. Vitamin C is possibly the most vital vitamin to the immune system. It has a direct effect on viruses and bacteria needed for creating adrenal hormones and lymphocytes.*

- *Vitamin E is working synergistically with other vitamins such as vitamin A and vitamin C, also the mineral selenium as the scavenger of toxic free-radicals.*

- *Zinc encourages healing of wounds and boosts the immune system response.*

- *Germanium is a trace element which helps the immune system.*

- *Get plenty of sleep.*

- *Avoid Smoking.*

- *Exercise Frequently*

- *Reduce stress and anxiety levels.*

Stress often triggers alterations in biochemistry that suppress white blood cell activity and overstretches the endocrine system in ways that can result in reduced defence against infection, and a reduced capability for healing. Stress depletes the body of its nutrients. Therefore tackling chronic stress is most important in getting the immune system back into balance.

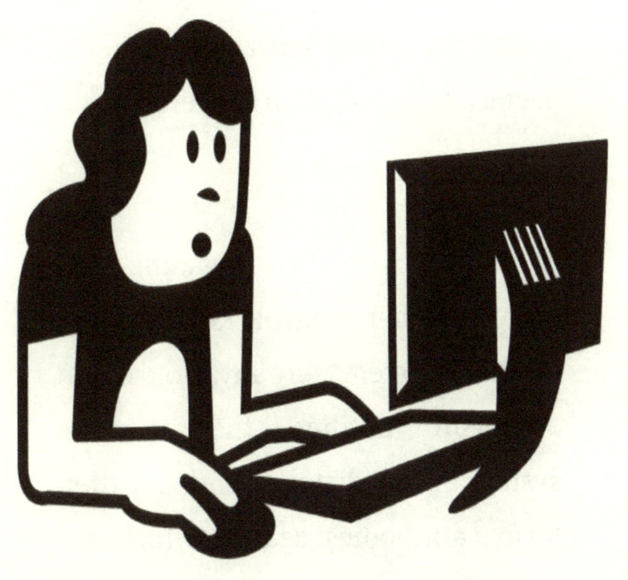

More Ways to Improve Your Immune System

The immune system has an incredible function in producing antibodies to combat any infections, bacterial, fungal, even cancer.

If a microorganism invading our body is under control, killed by the immune system; any invasion by an organism notifies the immune system immediately, and it then forms antibodies against whichever organism to destroy it.

There are several forms of immune system issues, and they separate into four categories:

1. *Immunodeficiency disorders can be primary or acquired. The primary immune deficiency disorder can be a deficiency that is the most common kind.*

2. *The second category is the autoimmune disorders whereby the immune system attacks its cells.*

3. *The immune system overreacts to an antigen, and*

*this kind comes under allergic
disorders.*

4. *The last and final type of
   immune system issue is the
   cancers of the immune
   system.*

Those with weak immune systems can take immunity boosters which can help to improve the immune system and result in the required antibodies, to fight off any infections.

Allopathic, herbal, and homoeopathic immunity boosters have been used to assist the immune system. There are several natural herbal medications around on the market:

- *Ashwagandha*
- *Echinacea*
- *Liquorice*
- *Siberian Ginseng*

Many food supplements mentioned earlier with Vitamin C and Vitamin E, and minerals such as Zinc, Iron, and Selenium improve the immune system too.

Food rich in vitamin C is citrus fruits; broccoli, green peppers, and cantaloupes. Also, whole grain foods; vegetable oils rich in Vitamin E, some meats, tofu, and dried beans have rich Iron content. Additionally, fish, nuts, and grains have rich selenium content.

Other ways of boosting your immune system would be getting more sun or taking vitamin D as a supplement which is quite efficient.

Also crucial to the immune system and general well-being:

- *do what you love*

- *Maintain good social relationships*

- *Have a positive outlook and attitude*

These are not necessarily boosters but healthy ways of being. If we become stressed, unhappy, depressed it affects our body as a whole; we become run down, depressed and more susceptible to catching germs like colds and the flu.

Bear in mind that you want your immune system to be well balanced, natural and healthy, not too boosted or hyper-vigilant.

Raising or boosting the immune system too much can also have adverse effects in making you feel weaker, sicker, as a result of your immune system battling any infection which is viral, and is often the sign of a healthy immune system.

Therefore, an imbalance in the immune system has the potential to develop into other types of inflammatory conditions, so always speak to a medical professional before you decide to boost your immunity.

Autoimmune Diseases

What Are Autoimmune Diseases?

Autoimmune diseases can appear baffling to most of us. The word autoimmune is an umbrella term that includes many different types of conditions. It also means that our immune system which is intended to protect us; fight against all kinds of invaders, bacteria etc. begins to turn on us, and attacks our healthy cells.

The connective tissue diseases are affecting our muscles, skin, nervous and connective tissue, our bones, blood and joints, even our body fat.

Because of the variety of organs and tissues etc. involved, it is why diagnosis can be complicated surrounding connective tissue, and why so many specialists are sometimes required, as in the case of Lupus, for example, this affects the kidneys, brain, and skin.

There are many system organs affected. Examples below:

- *Rheumatoid Arthritis (RA) connective tissue disease joints, leading cause of disability.*

- *Sjogren's Destruction of the glands that tears, dry eyes and mouth saliva.*

- Type 1 Diabetes insulin
  pancreas.

- Crohns – intestinal system.

- MS is attacking the nervous
  system.

- Psoriasis the body attacks its
  skin.

- Vasculitis blood vessels
  attacked.

- Thyroid or Hashimoto's
  disease the body attacks the
  thyroid.

Here are a few more:

- *VKH rare*
- *Necrobiosis Lipoidica*
- *ITP immune thrombocytopenia low or no platelets*
- *Goodpasture's Syndrome*
- *Raynaud's syndrome*
- *Alopecia (hair follicles)*
- *Graves' disease*
- *Ankylosing spondylitis*
- *Polymyalgia rheumatic or PMR*
- *Fibromyalgia*
- *Vasculitis*
- *PBC primary biliary cholangitis (liver)*
- *Sarcoidosis*
- *Lyme*
- *Celiacs disease*

- *Lichen planus*
- *Neurosarcoidosis*
- *Transverse Myelitis Awareness*
- *MCTD*

Please note that Epstein Bar and HIV are viruses and not an autoimmune disease.

Nature (genetics) and Nurture (environment)

It appears that there are genetic links and environmental triggers related to autoimmune diseases.

Boosting the Immune System – the last thing you should do?

Autoimmune diseases are conditions whereby your immune system is misguidedly attacking your own body so if it were possible to "boost your immune system," so an essential and critical question to ask yourself is - wouldn't boosting your immune system be the last thing you wanted to do?

Consider the fact that most autoimmune diseases respond well to cortisone, which is used to dampen the immune response.

There are people whose immune systems do not work so for them, there are treatments to improve their immune function, but they do that by replacing something that is missing.

If you are not missing anything, then having more of it will not do you any good. In theory, something that could boost the immune system could increase the risks of autoimmune disease.

Autoimmune diseases represent inadequate control of immune responses. Start, continue, and stop. These are the three critical control steps for an immune response.

The way we currently understand it, an accurately controlled immune response starts when it should, continues long enough to restore homeostasis to the tissue/organ/body, and stops when the goals achieved.

So, it is essential to speak to a professional before boosting your immune system especially if you already have a condition or disorder.

Are You Really What You Eat?

What does this mean - you are what you eat? We recognise this headline from the past, yet it is right for the majority of us in this age of fast food, quick takeaways providing us with the wrong foods that we really ought to avoid eating if we want to be healthy. Just what do you need to do is eat all-natural nourishment that will boost your immune system.

Do we consume enough foods that contain anti-oxidants? Alternatively, do we recognise what anti-oxidants do for our health and wellness?

Antioxidants help to protect our systems versus the dreadful impacts that free radical molecules carry our body's healthy cells. Connected to premature ageing as well as an entire spectrum of diseases such as eye problems, cancer cells, and cardiovascular disease; they might also be the source of a few autoimmune disorders.

You will undoubtedly see that antioxidants are essential to our health and a way of living. The body generates antioxidants as a regular part of power production from the nutrition that we consume daily. Nevertheless, revealed to the results of smoking cigarettes, contamination, and chemicals in what we consume. However, these sorts of things boost the manufacturing of cost-free radicals.

What can we do to get over these impacts?

The solution is simple, that is to somehow or other increase the degree of antioxidants generated in the body, to overcome the added free radicals produced. Simply put, we need to improve your body immune system.

Without getting technological, the most effective way to do this is by consuming lots of plant foods and ensuring that your diet plan is full of these wholesome foods.

There are lots of anti-oxidants available in various fruits, nuts, veggies, beans, grains, and seeds.

You also need plant food consumption; red, yellow, orange, green; this will certainly ensure that you have a general balance of the anti-oxidants required by your body.

Some of the anti-oxidants that are very easy to get in their all-natural form are:

Vitamin E

Vitamin E found in avocado, nuts, seeds, wholegrain, and wheat bacterium; this could help with cardiovascular problems.

Lycopene

Found in red or pink fruits or veggies like tomatoes, these aids in avoiding cold sores, prostate cancer, and it may even aid to prevent skin cancer.

Lutein

Discovered in eco-friendly leafy vegetables, broccoli, cabbage lettuce; they aid to avoid cataracts, macular degeneration, and also other eye conditions.

Sulfur Compounds

These compounds found in garlic and onions, broccoli, cabbage and Brussel sprouts.

There are significant antioxidant benefits that can be obtained from broccoli if eaten the correct means.

Broccoli has a rich source of antioxidants, but if you grow salad sprouts from broccoli seeds as well as taste them in your salad, they include about thirty times extra antioxidants compared to broccoli consumed in the typical method. That will certainly aid your body to get a boost to your body immune system.

There are numerous foods you can eat, and this is not a complete list, but it will undoubtedly help you to create the anti-oxidants; there are thousands more, but this will provide an idea of where to start should you want to improve your health.

Detox and Diets

Can Your Liver Burn Fat Automatically?

The main feature of the liver is to transform food to power, as well as generate chemicals and enzymes required to melt fat.

Liver stores iron reserves, minerals and vitamins and also make bile to digest food. It additionally makes cholesterol. It filters and purifies alcohol, medicines, reserves energy or sugar, as well as removes the toxins including the toxins that you breathe.

Your liver is a crucial organ responsible for the breakdown of fat.

The unfortunate reality is that a very high percentage of obese people have malfunctioning livers.

The liver generates bile, a result of blood filtering system. Bile transports from the liver, and stored in the gallbladder.

When fats consumed, the gallbladder releases bile to emulsify the fat right into tiny beads. Without bile, fat digestion is impossible. Considering that the liver is the vital body organ for fat digestion the liver needs to be in good condition if you want to lose fat.

You can look after your liver in the
following way:

- *Avoid unnecessary medicines.*

- *Avoid or limit alcohol.*

- *Never mix alcohol with
  medication or other
  medication.*

- *Avoid sugary treats, desserts,
  and drinks.*

- *Wear a mask over your
  mouth when using aerosol
  cleaners, if possible.*

- *Increase your consumption of
  high-fibre foods like fresh
  fruits and vegetables, bread,
  grains, rice and cereals.*

- Avoid using steroids because creates fatty liver.

If you need a natural remedy for revitalising the liver, Aloe Vera is something to try. Aloe Vera is known for rejuvenating the cells of the liver.

Aloe Vera is known worldwide for the cosmetic industry for invigorating skin cells. Ayurveda specialists have utilised the same cell rejuvenating property of Aloe Vera in India for a long time.

Aloe Vera is a plant from the lily plant group that grows up to 2-3 feet tall. This plant grows primarily in warm environments.

The gel in the leaves utilised for internal consumption. Aloe Vera gel supplies the nutrients needed by the internal organs of the body and speeds up the healing process.

It consists of the following nutrients:

- *Vitamin B12*
- *Vitamin C*
- *Vitamin E*
- *Beta-carotene*

Enzymes assists in digesting the food. It includes 20 essential Amino acids required by the body as a necessary foundation for healthy protein.

Minerals such as:

- *Iron*
- *Manganese*
- *Potassium*
- *Calcium*
- *Chromium*
- *Copper*
- *Zinc*
- *Magnesium*

- Consists of powerful *anti-inflammatory agents* called plant sterols.

- Includes Lignin, this is a woody compound which permits Aloe to pass through the skin.

- The salicylic acid in Aloe acts as an *anti-inflammatory* which aids to break down the dead tissues.

- Also, contains natural pain relievers referred to as Anthraquinones. Saponins are the soapy substances which have antimicrobial activity.

Aloe Vera strengthens the body's immunity and eliminates all the sludge, and waste material from areas of the bowel and liver. It provides the liver with all the needed nutrients and manages its functioning as well as repairs it from inside. Once the liver starts its normal function, fat dissolves automatically.

Herbal Detoxification

- *Are you overweight or worn out regularly?*

- *Do you have migraines, various other pains, and discomforts?*

- *How about frequent colds and cases of influenza?*

- *Do you have bowel irregularity or gastrointestinal problems?*

- *Maybe hypertension?*

- *Suffer from severe PMS*

- *What about allergic reactions or sensitivities?*

- *Do you drink too much alcohol, drink caffeinated drinks?*

- *Do you smoke cigarettes?*

- *Use non-prescription or leisure medicines?*

- *Do you eat your food too quickly?*

- *Do you eat fried or processed frozen foods?*

I am sure we can all answer yes to one of these questions.

Precisely what is a detox?

Our bodies have an all-natural built-in detoxification system comprised of the absorb tract; the urinary system, and the liver, that helps to refine all the chemicals contemporary life throws at it. These chemicals or 'contaminants,' and they are primarily poisons that have hazardous impacts on your body. It is not just alcohol and cigarettes full of toxic substances; pesticides and food additives, high levels of caffeine and also air pollution can all play their role too.

Advantages of a detoxification diet plan

1. Detoxification diet plans are believed to protect against persistent diseases, such as joint inflammation, heart problem, and also cancer cells.

2. People that attempt a detoxification diet usually find it could boost toxicity symptoms such as exhaustion, joint pain, headache, discomfort, premenstrual syndrome, undesirable skin, inadequate focus, stress and anxiety as well as impatience, constant colds, heartburn, constipation, as well as flatulence.

3. Detoxification diet plans suggested as part of a supervised treatment for persistent conditions such as autoimmune illnesses. Additionally, multiple chemical levels of sensitivity, fibromyalgia, chronic fatigue syndrome, digestive system problems, cardiovascular disease, and joint inflammation.

Detoxification Hot Tips

1. Clear the detox duration period in your journal of any bars, clubs, dining establishments, as well as events. See it as a chance to do all those things you never get around to, such as visiting museums and galleries, and after that, you could feel twice as smug at the end of it when you are not only healthier but more cultured too.

2. Drink water to prevent dehydration.

3. Take milk thistle to enhance these advantages; it has silymarin, which secures the liver from damage.

Mind-Body Detox

Unique chiropractic care therapies for addictions have been successful in stabilising those withdrawing from medications, and also another addictive behaviour. A Mind-Body Detox recognised by the clinical as well as medical professionals and even their magazines worldwide.

Addicts desiring to conquer their addiction is seeking practitioners utilising activator approaches to treat inadequate wellness, pain, and even addiction. The mind-body detoxification process triggers motion delicately, promoting the mind's enjoyment receptors as well as influences feelings in a positive method.

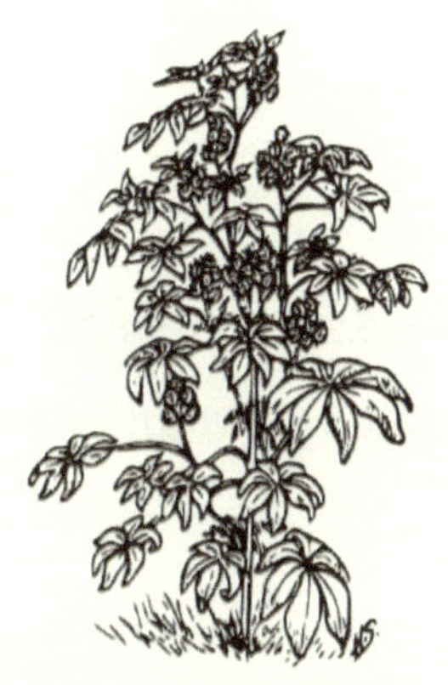

Astragalus

An antioxidant defending the liver from toxins, and strengthens the immune system. It generates anticancer cells in the body.

Echinacea

Improves lymphatic function and enhances the immune system.

Gingko Biloba

This antioxidant increases circulation to the brain cells.

Goldenseal

Antibacterial boosts the immune system, cleansing the blood. Do not take internally for over a week at a time or if pregnant.

St. John's Wort

A blood purifier is useful for incidences of HIV and Epstein - Barr virus.

Olive Leaf

Olive leaf has been useful against bacteria, fungi, and viruses. Treated with Epstein-Barr disease; AIDS or HIV, Herpes and Chronic Fatigue Syndrome.

Spirulina

Spirulina assists in with the protection of immune system and in eliminating toxins from the body. Technically, known as nutrient instead of a herb, spirulina, digestible natural food can protect the immune system and helps with mineral absorption. It assists in balancing the blood sugar levels and nutrients supplies which help the body heal and cleanse itself.

Other herbs that boost the immune response are:

- Bayberry
- Hawthorn
- Horehound
- Fenugreek
- Red Clover

Herbal Formulas

Herbs very often work for the better if used in combination with a selection of other herbs. However, there may be contradictions with some herbs if you have an auto-immune disorder. Do check with a proper herbal specialist or herbalist to create a blend that will be appropriate for your requirements.

Cleansing the Liver

Our liver is the primary purifying organ, and it needs to be functioning at its best for good immunity protection.

Black Radish, Dandelion, and Milk Thistle are herbs which are known to be useful for cleansing the liver.

The Best Ways to Select a Herbal Detox Diet Plan

Contaminants can include fragrance, alcohol, cigarette smoke, pesticides, mercury, artificial additive, contraceptive pills, and also cleansing materials. Toxins are transformed chemically to much less harmful substances secreted in stools or urine.

Consult your healthcare centre to find out if a detox diet plan is right for you. A detox diet plan must not be undergone by pregnant or nursing women, children, or individuals with anaemia, eating disorders, heart problems, reduced immunity, reduced high blood pressure, abscess, diabetic issues, epilepsy, cancer, or ulcerative colitis unless suggested and supervised by your primary care centre.

There are countless detoxification strategies you could follow, so select carefully. Some will undoubtedly support full fasting or juice-only days, but beware of the health effects and never begin any extreme strategy without consulting your medical professional or a certified nutritional expert.

Detoxification Advantages

1. Enhances symptoms of heartburn, irregularity, and gas as well as treats digestive problems;

2. encourages the body immune system.

Allergic reactions or sensitivities?

Typically, standard health care manages to mask the signs of allergies and food sensitivities, instead of trying to resolve them.

Elimination

The very first step that many different specialists advise is a modification of diet plan that eliminates wheat as well as milk foods; two common allergens found. To do so is the very first step in "detoxing." Higher levels of detoxing, in addition to extra immune support via nutritional supplementation have been recognised to help several allergy victims. Allergic reactions are, however, a very individualised condition.

Exactly what takes place after the detoxification?

A few of the foods eliminated during this diet can be allergenic. A natural health expert could assist in reintroducing specific food groups systematically such as wheat, dairy products, gluten, corn. Then note any reactions you may have, to identify the food groups that may be aggravating your health and wellness problems, such as sinus congestion, tiredness, skin conditions, arthritis as well as bloating and also bowel irregularity. Flare-ups can happen, so guidance highly recommended.

Taking Care of Your Colon

Incidences of cancer appear to be on the rise. Colon cancer, like heart disease, is taken into consideration a twentieth-century illness, as it was unusual before the very early 1900s. Many professionals consider colon cancer to be directly related to what you eat.

Taking better care of your colon and minimising the danger of colon problems or cancer can be accomplished by modifications in your diet, exercise routine, and way of living. Of the 3, food is one of the most essential.

Lack of fibre in the diet plan is the leading source of colon issues. Fibre assists the colon to operate efficiently. By merely including more bread and vegetables to your diet plan can help keep your colon doing its work and enable your bowels to empty on a regular basis. Soy items, as well as raised calcium intakes, have likewise been linked to favourable colon health and wellness.

Water is, of course, essential to all parts of the body, however particularly vital in forming correct faeces and colon elimination. The eight glasses still apply to today. Soy products, as well as various other calcium-rich foods, can be beneficial to colon health and wellness and well being.

Working out is vital to colon health and wellness. Regular exercise, also simple walking, aids the colon by permitting the toxic substances to continue to move through the body. Inactive lifestyles contribute to colon problems.

The wrong things you can do to your colon is waiting to pass the faeces when you feel need 'to go.' By not allowing your body to work, as it needs to, the wastes back up in the colon as well as begins to decay. Refraining from going to the bathroom can also result in either irregularity or diarrhoea, depending upon the contaminants in the stool. By without delay discharging the faeces as needed, the body frees itself of the toxins and also, keeps the colon and even the whole tract healthy.

Reducing the dangers of colon problems could limit the threats of other incapacitating illnesses such as appendicitis. Good colon wellness can also prevent dietary deficiencies. Any signs of irregular bowel movements or diarrhoea taken seriously and even if they linger, should be gone over with your physician instantly.

Goji Berries A Super Food

We all heard the term "superfood" right? Do you know what it implies? Superfoods are health foods considered beneficial owing to their health-protecting qualities. Therefore, to be certified as a superfood, you need to be abundant in the necessary antioxidants, fas, vital amino acids, etc. similar to that of Goji berries.

We cannot dismiss that Goji berries are abundant with different health benefits and their dietary values. This fruit includes 18 amino acids with high quantities of vitamins A, C, E, B1, B2, and B6. Also, it is rich in iron, anti-oxidants lutein, phytonutrient, zeaxanthin and 21 other essential minerals.

Unique compounds such as Lyciumbarbarum polysaccharides are even found in Goji berries, that are important in improving the immune system. Implemented by way of Goji berries packed with polysaccharides, offers the immune system cells with the particular sugars to enhance their interaction.

Simultaneously, polysaccharides provide energy permanently. The intestinal tract bacteria works applicably and helps in boosting the body immune system.

As these nutrients help in sustaining the immune and probiotic cells of the body; the immune system kept healthy which helps reduce inflammation in the various components of the body. Currently, Goji berries utilised as medicines for inflammation-based conditions like bronchial asthma, pain, allergies, cancer and so forth. Likewise, it is made use of in autoimmune problems such as rheumatoid arthritis; Crohn's disease, and even lupus as a result of the polysaccharides found in Goji berries. The nutrient Polysaccharides protects the liver from severe damage during extreme body exercise workouts.

In summary, there are many health benefits in Goji berries. It can act as a sex or libido booster too, described as a natural Viagra. It improves general well being and enhances cellulite as Goji berries have anti-oxidants that are healthy for the skin.

Other benefits of Goji berries

- *reduces the ageing process*
- *helps with weight-loss*
- *combats cancer cells*
- *combats heart diseases*
- *boosts hearing*
- *boosts vision*
- *acts as a fertility enhancer*
- *builds muscle mass*
- *strengthens bones, ligaments*
- *cleanses the liver and kidneys*

□

These are a few benefits of Goji berries, and why Goji berries are considered a superfood. However, although these superfoods thought about healthy and balanced for the body, we need to bear in mind that our diet plan needs to not consist just of these foods alone. We still have to stick to what's healthy, and that is through adhering to a well-balanced diet regimen that includes the intake of fruits, veggies, low-fat milk products, slim, healthy proteins and also high fibre foods.□

Organic Foods

As you could see, the advantages of health foods are numerous. There are many benefits, however, what are the benefits of organic foods? Well, to start with, health foods are produced as though there are no chemicals in the growing process.

No chemicals are introduced into the mix as well as only natural fertilisers, chemicals, or herbicides used. In the case of farm animals, organic feed to them, so you can be assured that you obtain organic meats or milk by subjective criteria.

There are also other benefits to health food which includes the exclusion of genetically modified organisms (GMO). GMO's to put it succinctly are foods which have had their genetic structure altered in some way or other.

While this may appear to yield numerous advantages in the field of agriculture by offering farmers with more significant amounts of useable plants, no one still totally understands what the negative aspects are of changing the genetic framework of living organisms. You have to look no further to find deficiencies that scientific research found out about years after regular and extensive use.

So to that level, the benefits of organic food much exceed the dubious goodness of non-organic foods. The only issue is the high price of organic foods, the expenses that you might have upon seeing your monthly food costs, after going all natural, may put you off the many benefits of organic food until they become to be more economical to buy.

Paleo Diet

Paleo diet plan or the Neanderthal diet regimen is a type of diet that is getting much popularity after its rediscovery. The Paleo diet plan has become one of one of the most sort after terms on the internet, and this alone is a sign that numerous individuals are fascinated by this new however old kind of diet regimen. If you are perplexed about it, then don't be.

The diet plan may sound like a brand-new fad diet, yet it is the diet regimen that our ancestors have been complying with, and it appeared to work for them.

When discovering Paleo diet regimen, it is best to submerge oneself in the characteristics of the diet. Supporters of paleo diet regimens claim that our forefathers are stronger and also did not experience any metabolic diseases that we have today. The diet plan added immensely on exactly how they have warded off problems and also stayed strong as they undergo their daily grind without much help with innovation and machinery that we have today.

The idea behind paleo diet is simple, eat what our forefathers had eaten as well as do the workload of our forefathers, and you will obtain a healthy and balanced body because of this. However, this is simpler said compared to done. While you will have the privilege of eating as much food as well as the type of food that each one would like to eat, you still need to work your butt off to make the food you eat work, to your advantage.

Confused? Here are some of the things that you should learn about the diet.

In the 1970s, the Paleo diet advocates recognised the work of Walter Voegtlin who introduced this principle many years ago. Voegtlin proposed that Paleolithic diet plan is better for humans, which genetics have almost changed even with the introduction of agriculture. Voegtlin said that the best diet regimen for people is the diet plan used by Paleolithic forefathers.

Today, this diet plan stays among the crucial debates with physicians and also dietitians. The Health Service of the United Kingdom rejects this diet regimen as a trend. Doubters said that the diet plan might cause possible health and wellness problems, as an unbalanced diet regimen could do even more harm than good.

Advocates of the diet plan say that people ought to return to eating the way our ancestors did because of the vast varieties of people that are overweight and obese that caused countless diseases.

The Paleo diet is taking advantage of the natural means of eating and also the designed diet regimen for humans. The menu will undoubtedly bring about better health as well as longer lives.

The Paleo diet eliminates sugar and also sugar from damaging the body. No grains included which it was not developed to consume. Also, no processed foods, considering that our ancestors had never processed or prepared treated food available. In fact, people with cancer had better lifespans with sugar eliminated from their diet.

The body has been using carbs as the principal resource of power. The proponents of paleo diet plan believe that the body is made to run at a low carbohydrate level. The body has a means to discover new resources of power, and it will consume the fat in the body with ketogenesis. When there is the lack of sugar, the body looks to body fat as a source of energy.

However, before you try this diet plan, it is best that you speak with a medical professional whether this sort of diet plan is acceptable for you. Despite Paleo diet regimen plan, your wellness and welfare are of vital importance, and a health professional could help you determine it.

Health Problems Solved by Paleo Diet

Paleo diet plan is not only excellent to slim down. The mechanics of the diet plan can likewise help individuals decrease dangers of particular conditions. The manner of picking the right food groups as consumed by our forefathers can unlock the enigma why there are disorders that exist today, which were absent before.

Paleo experts think that a lot of the illnesses that exist today linked to the type of foods that we eat today. The foods that we eat have lots of sugar as well as salts that might trigger a great deal of illness. Eliminating some of the foods by sticking to a paleo diet regimen can help people alleviate some of the risks and ultimately live longer and fuller lives.

Diabetes mellitus

The elimination of sugars and also specific grains from the diet will help lower the blood glucose degrees as well as preserve it. Diabetic issues are a persistent disease that could harm the kidney, eyes or even bring about amputations. People shed arm or legs as a result of gangrene as a result of poor blood circulation as part of the wellness risks positioned by diabetes mellitus.

Diabetes is the result of inadequate sugar absorption in the body. The body often creates insulin resistance where the insulin does not correctly process the sugar because of a variety of factors. Diabetes mellitus patients could obtain a great deal of aid from a paleo diet regimen since it decreases the sugar absorption. The much less sugar implies there would undoubtedly be reduced blood sugar degrees.

High blood pressure

Hypertension can be aggravated by eating excessive salt. One of the aspects of the paleo diet plan is the non-consumption of processed foods. Refined foods commonly have great deals of salt which keeps water.

When the body retains extra water, it offers the body a harder time to reduce the high blood pressure. Although there is a debate whether a paleo diet can bring high blood pressure down as a result of boosted cholesterol consumption, there is yet a robust research study to profess that cholesterol without a doubt causes high blood pressure. There is indeed a further reason high blood pressure exists, and the cholesterol degrees are simple spectators that may add to the situation. The writing remains on the wall as the court is still out whether high cholesterol and if there is without a doubt a difference between dietary cholesterol and also blood cholesterol.

Immune system boost

One of the troubles of the body is its failure to take care of inflammation. Swelling is one of the reasons the immune system is getting impaired. A damaged immune system indicates that the body is more susceptible to microbes as well as infections. The boosted usage of Omega 3 fatty acids assists the body battle against inflammation and indirectly help increases the immune system.

Acne

Acne is one of the most unexpected illnesses that are being attended to by a paleo diet plan. The rise in Omega 3 fats along with probiotics, anti-oxidants, and selenium can help regulate the inflammation and also to eliminate the germs that can cause acne. Acne is not uncommon to people as 80 percent will undoubtedly suffer some degree of acne when in their lives.

There are lots of health advantages in eating paleo. It is necessary that you can seek advice from a paleo diet-friendly physician to offer you the very best alternatives and much better discuss with you the benefits as well as the mechanics of the paleo diet. It is a revolutionary means of dropping weight, and it could help you over time.

The Paleo Diet Basics

Maybe you have heard of some individuals "eating like cavemen" and shiver to assume just what type of foods they eat. That is unfair to quickly wrap up that Paleo diet is eating like a crude cave dweller.

Firstly, exactly what does Paleo diet regimen mean? The word paleo originates from words Paleolithic that ended for around 10000 earlier. It is called Paleo because of the foods or let us claims the way of living in this sort of diet regimen usually found throughout the Paleolithic era. It is also known as the diet plan of seeker gatherer, caveman, or the stone-age civilisation; the significant concepts of this diet plan based on its name. During this period, people would typically eat foods that are common to them. These foods are fish, nuts, veggies, fruits like berries and also seeds. Scientists today after that think about individuals during the Paleolithic era stable and even healthy; they were regarded fit to handle the devastations of those times.

It allowed them to walk around often and also for extended periods. Paleo individuals discovered how to not have conditions such as cancer, heart troubles, or excessive weight. They are in shape and full of energy. Do you understand the reasons behind that? Naturally, that is because of the type of food they eat and way of life they had.

If you are into Paleo diet, the foods that you eat are vegetables mainly the origin veggies except or potatoes or perhaps the beautiful potatoes. The diet plan is composed a lot of fruits, almonds, as well as walnuts as sole food or active ingredients in the Paleo dishes. You could likewise include peanuts in addition to cashews in your diet regimen.

For some, they go for berries like raspberries, strawberries, and blueberries because of its performance that lots of people currently showed it. While there are foods that you should not eat, foods like parsnips, carrots, rutabagas, or the body organ meats such as kidneys and also liver increased.

If you are a person that is in diet regimen mainly this Paleo diet one, you should not eat pasta, string beans, noodles, bread, snow-peas, milk items as well as sugar. This is the routine that you need to adhere to when in diet such this. When you get up during the morning, you scramble some eggs then you could fruit together with the yoghurt. You can likewise include coffee or tea to your dish and also have a little amount of milk on it. For your lunch, you could have with you a tossed salad with dressing on it. Finally, for your supper have a rejuvenating and mouth-watering barbequed fish, steak, or poultry with environment-friendly veggies of your selection.

The checklist of foods offered right here is all low in carbohydrates yet higher in healthy protein given that all the carbs that you are most likely to consume are all from vegetables. Moreover, you have to need an animal fat because this would be the primary resource for your power.

For those wondering if the Paleo diet is healthy and also efficient, well, the solution is yes. However, why? Paleo diet plan includes trimming unnatural foods or the processed foods overcooked. Individuals on this diet regimen would indeed just quit absorbing way too many carbs and would certainly just rely on fats or healthy proteins to keep them going. If you are dedicated sufficient to this sort of diet plan, time will certainly tell that your food cravings for salted foods and desserts will merely stop.

You ought to make note initially that when you are into the type of diet plan, don't be too warm in attaining the sort of body fit you want. However, one thing is for sure you could have the result that you wish in an issue of time. You merely should adhere to the Paleo diet plan program.

The Trouble Low Carb/High Healthy Protein Diets

Do they function? Yes, you do lose weight initially on a High Protein/Low Carb diet plan however 90% of your initial weight-loss is water.

Just what takes place after your body has dropped its water weight? It starts to burn the leftover fat and then because it lacks carbs to melt for power, it begins to shed protein - your muscular tissues. These diet regimens induce a metabolic condition called ketosis which is an annoying problem found in people who experience kidney illness as well as diabetes, not typically found in healthy people. Burning protein is not healthy and balanced since healthy protein is nature's structure material and is crucial for fixing and restoring your body's cells, tissues and also body organs. Supporters of the Low Carb/High Protein/Fat diets downplay ketosis as well as case its evidence your body's burning fat. That is true in part. Ketosis does melt fat yet will indeed likewise, eventually; burn your body's muscle cells.

If you have ever gotten on among these diet regimens, you have observed that your pee gets yellow. This results from ketones which are a by-product of ketosis. This is evidence that your body is melting and separating muscle mass cells which is protein. That is dangerous since if excessive of your body's healthy protein is broken down, you could endure irreparable liver and kidney damages. More symptoms of muscle mass failure appear in general weak point, fatigue and also the absence of power.

One more thing to think about Low Carb/High Protein diet plans is that during the process of ketosis your body likewise breaks down fats and also converts them to ketones and also acetones which used for gas. An adverse effect of this is that your body sheds essential minerals like potassium as well as sodium. This decreases your thyroid hormone degree which then reduces your metabolic process and also ultimately your price of fat burning. Additionally, ketosis might increase your blood cholesterol degrees which are indeed not a risk-free scenario.

When you quit the diet plan the weight piles right back on, and there are an essential means to prevent this. Do not limit your diet plan to anyone food team or group.

As opposed to blindly cutting Carbohydrates and also increasing protein and fat consumption, you need to opt for a healthy and balanced ratio of 30% healthy protein, 15% fat, and 55% complex carbohydrates. This proportion will aid you to slim down gradually as well as securely. The trick is to decrease fat as well as simple carbs, not carbohydrates in general.

Another downside of low carb/ high-Fat diets is that studies show that the fewer carbs you indulge in, the more likely you will eat more fat; besides excess fat accumulated in your body's fat cells, where they will remain indefinitely, blocking your arteries with unhealthy cholesterol. Therefore, the more fat you eat, the more your body will undoubtedly retain despite how little carbohydrates you consume, even if you eat no carbs whatsoever.

Currently here's the secret concerning consuming complex carbohydrates. Because complex carbs have a low glycaemic index, your body needs to burn 250% more energy to convert these carbs into fuel compared, to transform fat into energy. Your body works harder to metabolise as well as melt calories from complex carbs, compared to High Protein/Low Carbs.

The outcome is safe, organised weight reduction, which means you stay clear of health problems, and sagging skin caused by quick weight loss.

The Gluten-Free Diet

I can tell you honestly that up until very recently I had little knowledge regarding what a gluten-free diet was. I had an idea that I might suffer from it myself. Nonetheless, gluten is just what you would call the protein part of certain grains like wheat, barley, rye or other comparable grains. Some people are found to be adverse to the gluten in these grains. Therefore, they should follow a gluten-free diet plan.

Unfortunately, that is not as very easy as it sounds. Moreover, since a person who deals with gluten intolerance or celiac illness has to live their whole lives on a gluten-free diet to be able to live an ordinary healthy and balanced life, they will need to talk to a medical professional or nutritional expert initially. If they do not obtain the diet regimen that's right for them, they could be facing numerous issues.

Should you suffer from these gluten allergic reactions, don't worry too much as there is hope. A diet plan that can suit your individual needs formulated and you can live a good life. Stay away from wheat-based items. Once more that may not be so simple, but with assistance, you can discover the best gluten-free diet for you.

If you like oats, then you will be glad to hear that you do not need to remove oats or oat items from your plan. If refined without the polluting agents of wheat or such various other grains, then you should be fine. However, make sure that is the case otherwise, you will undoubtedly be unintentionally having gluten into your system.

Foods that you could consume on your gluten-free diet could consist of corn, soy, rice, as well as pudding. You have selections of jams, as well as marmalades, sugar, honey, antidote, and molasses as well. If that is insufficient, your gluten-free diet could include all fresh vegetables and fruits, also eggs, milk, creams, types of butter and cheeses. You can have tea and coffee, carbonated beverages and alcoholic drinks too.

Although it may not be that straightforward to stay on your gluten-free diet, if you begin buying all kinds of prepared foods, these might consist of items with gluten in them. As well as if not real gluten based products they may have been processed somewhere near where there are gluten based products.

So, if you stay on the fresh side of your food, as well as steer clear of from canned or ready-made items, after which all you need is your gluten-free product. Together with this, you must stay away from anything that has wheat or suchlike as this could ruin your gluten-free diet plan. With some preparation, you will be fine, and your diet should remain intact.

Speed Up Metabolism & Lose Weight Naturally

The diet industry is a multi-million dollar sector and, of course, there are those firms that profit from this market. So, if there was a checklist of foods that could speed up your metabolic process and help you to reduce weight efficiently, the diet plan industry will not want you to learn about it.

What happens if that list of foods consisted of the type of foods that you love to consume? Is that possible? Would it be breaking the diet plan regulations which would not allow it? Nevertheless, do not all diet plans inform you to eliminate those foods that you like the most? You must only consume low-fat foods and stay clear of things like nuts and also grains. You should stay away from healthy and balanced vegetables and fruits because they consist of too much all-natural sugar - right?

Wrong!

If all these fad diets were appropriate to consume low-fat foods, eat low-carb foods, eat protein only, eat cabbage soup until it comes out your ears and yet, after that why are obesity numbers still increasing?

The diet professionals available have no idea, or if they do know, they typically aren't informing you, if so, they will make you pay a significant cost for the details. People spend hundreds of dollars to lose weight on the latest fat burning fad, so use sound judgment.

Whatever type of diet you are on; the bottom line is that you have to burn more calories than you eat. Common sense will tell you that if you keep your calorie consumption within a healthy and balanced range plus you do some exercise, you will drop in weight. There steps you can take to make slimming more straightforward, and that is to have a healthy diet regimen, and this consists of eating foods that offer your metabolism an increase which helps you to shed calories much faster.

Some foods high on the checklist of foods that accelerate metabolic rate are:

- *Tuna*
- *Salmon*
- *Sardines*

These foods are fantastic sources of Omega-3 fatty acids as well as heart-healthy fat, and they additionally assist in reducing your levels of leptin. When your leptin hormones stay in a reduced array, it is a lot easier to lose weight. So eating more fish will undoubtedly help to drop weight much faster. If you do not like fish, you can always take some fish oil supplements instead.

Olive oil is another excellent resource for Omega-3 and monounsaturated fats to improve metabolic process.

A few other weight loss foods are the warm and spicy kinds:

- *Cayenne*
- *Habanero*
- *Jalapeno peppers*

These peppers include capsaicin which is the compound that makes them hot; it is likewise the compound that provides your metabolic rate with a considerable increase for approximately three hours after you eat. To obtain the most of it, take advantage of these fat loss foods. You can choose tasty lower-fat, good carbohydrate, spicy recipes.

Entire grains are likewise excellent for accelerating the metabolic rate because they have a slow-moving food digestion rate and they maintain your blood sugar levels also.

Cinnamon

Cinnamon is one more food that has blood sugar controlling effects and could keep your metabolism going for longer.

After that, there are the protein-rich foods like:

- *Eggs*
- *Nuts*
- *Lean meats*
- *Pulses, beans*

These all offer your body the much-needed protein to keep it running smoothly.

Water, although a drink and not food, will also help in keeping your metabolic rate above speed. When losing weight, it is essential to maintain the advised day-to-day consumption of water to support your body at peak efficiency.

Forget all the brand-new crash diet, just alter your diet a little to consist of several of these very metabolic process foods, and include some exercise in your routine, and drink lots of water. You will begin to observe a difference in your weight efficiently and rapidly.

Stress and the Immune System

Anxiety or stress and the body immune system play an essential role in your life as well as total health. Every day, demanding events influence how your body responds to fighting illnesses. Difficult occasions that happen on a short-term basis can change the way your immune systems react momentarily.

Reactions from the immune system to temporary tensions could be valuable in many cases; positively redistributing cells to assist your body in adapting as a quick-fix. Moderately tricky situations, nevertheless, can have a harmful impact on your body's immune system, while distressing, as well as persistent, stress and anxiety, could compromise your immune system's capability to function properly.

Individuals respond in a different way to demanding situations: some experience more physiological modifications when under pressure compared to others. Anxiety and also the body immune system can bring about conditions where your body's cells could be subdued and made incapable of taking part in their useful features of shielding your body against infections.

From giving a demanding presentation in public to the usual traffic congestion that can turn into road rage, tension and the immune system play a substantial function in your overall wellness. If your body's immune system is not operating correctly, all sorts of bacteria, microorganisms, infections, and illness can enter your system to trigger off much more despair.

Bronchial asthma, diabetes, cardiovascular disease, and abscesses, are several of the conditions made worse by the effects of anxiety and also the immune system. Boosts in chemicals produced by your body that assist with nerve conduction cause adjustments in your heart rate as well as the capillary, compromising the immune system's feedback when you enter into scenarios that trigger your stress.

To assist in reducing the opportunities that stress, anxiety and the immune system adversely influence your everyday life, you can take action such as eating properly, obtaining routine exercise and more rest.

Your body needs your support to deal, assist and take care of you. Eating healthy and nourishing foods is an excellent way to start. The intake of foods such as orange vegetables; carrots, pumpkin, squash, and potatoes, all help with the Vitamin A that your skin needs to stop bacteria from entering into your body. Lean, low-fat beef, as well as particular types of mushrooms consisting of zinc, promote the structure of white blood cells to assist or battle the infection. Yoghurt, tea, and fortified cereals all help in keeping your body immune system operating well.

Likewise, you can try to lessen your stress levels to a minimum and try to practice deep-breathing exercises and various other tension calming techniques, to try to decrease stress. Tension, as well as the immune system, can negatively influence your body's health, wellness, and well-being once anxiety gets out of hand. Your body immune system is not up doing the necessary work. Stress is a physical process, yet you could take mindful actions to regulate it and get control over the circumstance before it going out of control, as well as preventing illness to ensure you.

Pressure is component all work and helps to keep us motivated. However, excessive anxiety can lead to stress, which undermines performance, is costly to employers and can make people ill.

Stress Assessments

In becoming stressed, people must, therefore, make two main assessments: firstly they must feel threatened due to the situation, and secondly, they must doubt that their capabilities and resources are sufficient to meet the threat.

Damaging Stress

How someone stressed feels about the potential damage he or she thinks the situation can cause them, and how adequate his or her resources meet the demands of the case. This sense of threat is rarely physical. It may, for instance, involve perceived risks to our social standing, to other people's opinions of us, to our career prospects or our own deeply held values.

Acute Stress

There are repercussions when the immune system acts in dispute or is exceptionally defensive.

1. The steroid hormones dampen parts of the immune system so that infection fighters; including white blood cells or other immune molecules, are redistributed.

2. These immune-boosting troops transported to the body's firing line whereby infection or injury is

probable, such as the skin, the lymph nodes, and bone marrow.

The Acute Response in the Mouth and Throat

Fluids get diverted from nonessential locations, including the mouth. The diversion will cause dryness in the mouth and difficulty in talking. Stress can also cause spasms of the throat muscles, making things difficult to swallow.

Stress Relief with a Stress Ball

When you squeeze a stress ball, the muscles contract in your hand and your arm. You can hold the squeeze ball for a second or two and release.

As your muscles relax, the tension leaves your arms and hands, relieving the stress. It is a beautiful way to take out your anger and frustration.

The Advantages of Massage Therapy

Massage therapy is all about touch. We are physical, and therefore our bodies respond well to massage therapy and human contact. When there is touch, more recovery happens.

These are a few of known health benefits of Massage Therapy:

1. Improves blood circulation, therefore enabling raised oxygen as well as nutrients to be delivered to treated locations consisting of locations that have been harmed or have experienced overexertion.

2. Helps to decrease high blood
    pressure.

3. Aids in detoxing by pushing
    toxic waste items with the
    lymphatic system.

4. Relieves tension and also
    promotes a sense of well
    being.

5. Relaxes injured muscle mass,
    minimising pains, and muscle
    spasms.

6. Stimulates the launch of the
    bodies' natural endorphins
    which could aid pain control.

7. Provides an enhanced body workout by stretching the skeletal muscles.

Evidence shows that massage therapy assists in reinforcing the body immune system of a person. Some research reveals changes in immune system following massage therapy, consisting of the new study on healthy women that show improvements in disease-fighting white blood cells, and all-natural killer-cell tasks.

Before a massage session, consult with the massage therapist about your therapy goals. Different mixes of massage therapy strategies could be made use of, to obtain these objectives. For example, if you have a sporting activities injury, you may want to have specific massage therapy strokes targeted to lower swelling and enhance blood flow in that location. Or the treatment session could merely be a necessary de-stressing and loosening up.

Do you agree that many of today's health problems are because of stress-related issues? Massage helps in the reduction of anxiety, and this can assist with white blood cells.

For a better immune system and reduced stress and anxiety levels, it may be worth your while to find out more about massage therapy.

As you have read in this last section, there are numerous autoimmune diseases, and it is essential to make sure you follow the right diet regime or detox, especially if you have an autoimmune disease, inflammatory condition or eating disorder.

There are plenty of beneficial foods you can eat. Emotional well-being is an essential component too and the less stress in your life the better. Easier said than done I know but there are ways you can manage your stress levels.

Other Autoimmune Diseases

Rheumatoid Arthritis

Rheumatoid arthritis affects one percent of the world's population. It is a persistent inflammatory disease, characterised by the inflammation of the lining, or synovium, of the joints. Rheumatoid arthritis is additionally an autoimmune illness, which indicates that the body immune system assaults regular tissue parts as if they were attacking the virus.

Rheumatoid arthritis swelling mainly attacks the linings of the joints. Nevertheless, the membrane layer cellular linings of the capillary, heart, as well as lungs, might also end up being inflamed.

The joints in the feet and hands are often affected by rheumatoid joint inflammation, but any joint lined by a membrane layer might be involved. Medication can regulate the swelling, redness, inflammation, soreness or defect in the joints results. This could lead to long-lasting joint damage, resulting in persistent pain, and special needs.

There are 3 phases of rheumatoid joint inflammation:

1. *The first stage begins with the swelling of the synovial lining, creating discomfort, warmth, rigidity, redness as*

well as swelling around the
joints.

2. The second stage is the rapid
    department as well as the
    growth of cells, or pannus,
    which triggers the enlarging
    of the synovium.

3. In the third phase, the
    inflamed cells releases
    enzymes that bone and also
    cartilage might soak up
    creating the included joint to
    even more discomfort,
    deformity as well as loss of
    activity.

Rheumatoid joint inflammation clients experience cycles of severe and also light signs. The adhering to are symptoms as well as effects of rheumatoid arthritis:

- *Joint swelling in smaller joints of the hands and even feet.*

- *Joint inflammation, rigidity, as well as discomfort especially in the early morning.*

- *Hardened lumps in joints.*

- *Cartilage material as well as the bone devastation.*

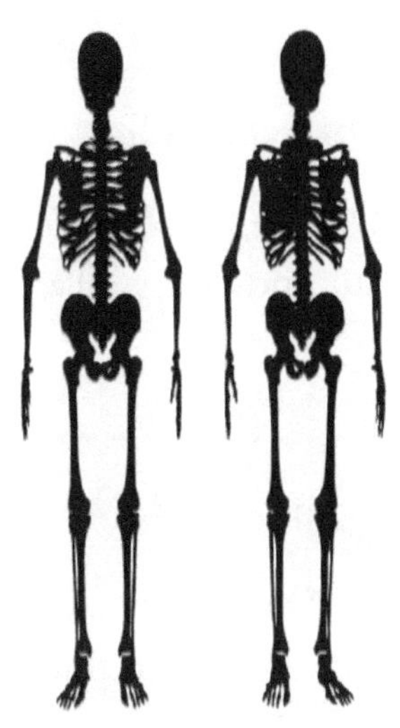

Rheumatoid joint inflammation can have a severe impact on a person's life, health, and wellness, especially if it is not discovered and dealt with early. Knowing the right diagnosis soon is crucial since it helps you to start the most suitable therapy quickly hence providing you with a better possibility to stay clear of impairment and deformity.

Consult your doctor about the diagnosis and also therapy of rheumatoid joint inflammation. With the correct diagnosis, you could take control of the disease with the best medication. Medical professionals have lots of ways to treat this disease, the goals of which is to remove pain, decrease swelling, decrease or quit joint damages, helps people feel much better, as well as help individuals, remain energetic.

Presently, the specific cause of the disease is unknown, although there are numerous ideas, like an irregular autoimmune response as discussed earlier or, genetic susceptibility, and again, some environmental aspects involved.

Scientists are well within their means to understanding the events that result in unbalanced responses of the body's body immune system. While there is no cure yet, regulating the disease with the use of brand-new medications, exercise, natural foods, and self-management methods, individuals have better, healthier and active lives.

Enjoy Life in Spite of Joint inflammation from Arthritis

Joint inflammation is a well-known joint problem that is recognised to create pain and also swelling to anybody that is unfortunate enough to get it. Arthritis caused by lots of things, such as age, joint injury, or autoimmune responses.

Home Appliances

Look into the Arthritis Foundation's listing of advised items and home appliances. There are plenty of devices that are not easy to open for someone that has arthritis, and there are particular home appliances that might be challenging to use. The checklist contains items and tools that can be used by a person with arthritis.

One way in which you could combat arthritis problems is to be in search of ergonomically-designed home tools. Today numerous suppliers generate home appliances and devices created to take full advantage of comfort and simplicity of use. Buying and using such items could help you avoid common anxiety as well as prevent joint inflammation flare-ups.

Apparently, using a walking stick when walking could alleviate up to twenty percent of your body weight off your legs and hips? This suggests you might minimise the pressure and stress on your legs while having the ability to move quickly. Ask your medical professional about walking canes and discover if it is right for you.

Vegan Diet

A study has shown that people with arthritis often have less discomfort, much less stiffness, as well as better grasp, strength than other individuals. If you are not ready to make this sort of adjustment, merely aim to consume more green foods. These foods could save you from tissue damage, which goes back to what you eat, it is crucial.

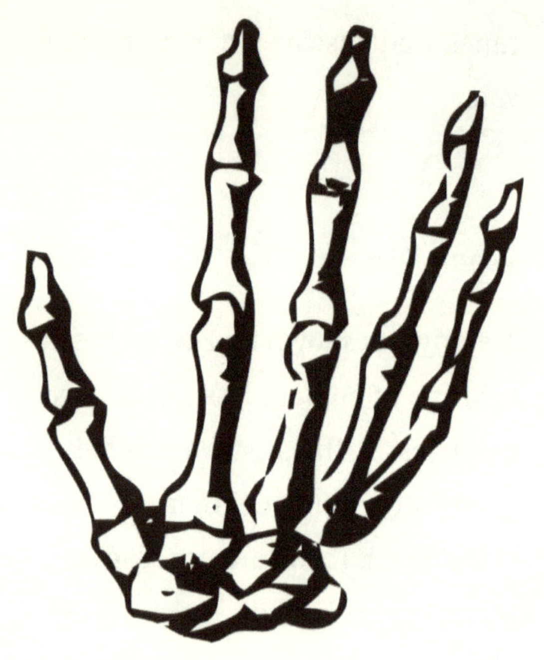

To handle your symptoms efficiently, perhaps attempt a Mediterranean diet plan. Researchers have shown that arthritis patients who use this diet plan see their symptoms quickly reduce, and they have a far better experience in general. The Mediterranean diet is high in healthy and balanced fats as well as grains, which your body uses for versatility and total wellness.

Exercise

Exercising is an excellent means to help minimise discomfort in the joints as well as tightness when having joint inflammation. Working out helps with weight, and difficult circumstances, provide more flexibility and helps individuals feel far better. You should choose workouts that are low impact, reduced effects. Swimming and strolling are great options for low impact exercises.

Plan your day wisely

You should do things when you have the energy to do them, and when your discomfort is low. Do not plan a hectic day if your arthritis troubles you often. Listen to your body, don't push it too far.

Support Group

Join a support group that includes other patients with joint inflammation. Friends, as well as relatives, may not always be encouraging of the discomfort you are in, or might just not recognise the crippling nature of the problem. Having group-buddies with joint inflammation could give you somebody to speak to about your discomfort, and won't judge you while taking the anxiety off of your family when aiming to handle your concerns.

In conclusion, any person who is unfortunate to have arthritis recognises that it causes unbearable pain and also inflammation in the joints. Once more, there are different causes for the condition, such as age, trauma, as well as autoimmune responses, each leading to a different sort of arthritis. Utilize these ideas to fight joint inflammation in your body.

Superfoods for Hives Alleviation

Hives referred to as urticaria, and they trigger increased white or yellow, scratchy wheals bordered by an area of red inflammation. It is an allergy to the skin, triggering the body to release histamine into the impacted cells. The dimension of the wheel itself varies, with the larger ones often joining together in position to form a bumpy rash. They usually cause severe inflammation as well as regularly appear on the arm or legs and also the trunk, but can occur anywhere. Intense urticaria develops swiftly and lasts for just as few hours - it is characterised by a burning or feverish, feeling as well as occasionally nausea. Chronic urticaria can continue for an extended period.

Common triggers include drugs such as aspirin as well as penicillin, artificial additive, food level of sensitivity such as milk eggs, shellfish as well as nuts, environmental variables such as direct exposure to cool, heat or sunlight, stress and anxiety and stress and anxiety, and also bites and also stings.

All vegetables and fruits consist of some amount of vitamin C.

Foods that tend to be the highest possible resources of vitamin C:

- *Green peppers*
- *Citrus fruits*
- *Fresh juices*
- *Strawberries*
- *Tomatoes*
- *Broccoli*
- *Turnip*
- *Eco-friendlies*
- *Leafy veg*
- *White potatoes*
- *Melon*
- *Spinach*

Vitamin C assists advertise a healthy and balanced immune system and also discharges antihistamines. Green tea has been reported to have an antihistamine outcome.

Vitamin B12 has been reported to minimise the intensity of severe hives as well as to reduce the frequency as well as the severity of episodes in persistent cases. Vitamin B12 found in animal foods, fortified foods, and also some fermented foods.

Some sources of B12 are:

- *Eggs*
- *Meat*
- *Fowl*
- *Fish*
- *Dairy products*
- *Foods made from soy*
- *Salmon*
- *Low-fat milk*

If you struggle with food allergies, it is essential to keep a comprehensive food diary. Note what you consumed when you have hives outbreaks, as it may be just a simple issue of eliminating the food or several foods from your diet plan to avoid struggling with hives.

Autoimmune Disorder Crohn's Disease

Crohn's condition is a systemic inflammatory digestive tract illness (IBD) for the unknown reason that results in chronic inflammation of the intestinal tract.

It could affect the entire stomach tract from mouth to anus, as well as could likewise cause issues beyond the stomach system.

The incidence of Crohn's condition in North America is 7:100 000, and is believed to be similar in Europe, however lower in Asia and Africa

Unlike the other primary inflammatory digestive tract condition, ulcerative colitis, there is no known medical or surgical cure for Crohn's illness.

Several clinical therapies are nonetheless available for Crohn's condition with a goal of maintaining the disease in remission.

Numerous individuals with Crohn's disease have symptoms for many years before the diagnosis. Due to the patchy nature of the intestinal illness as well as the deepness of tissue involvement, preliminary signs can be a lot more unclear than with ulcerative colitis.

Usual initial signs and symptoms of Crohn's illness consist of the adhering to abdominal pain, diarrhoea, bloody diarrhoea, and also a perirectal pain.

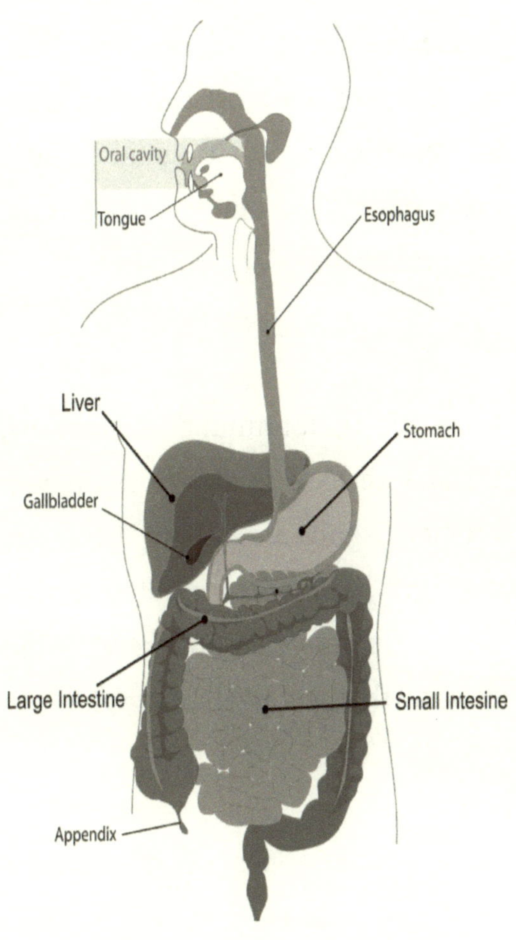

Oral cavity
Tongue
Esophagus
Liver
Stomach
Gallbladder
Large Intestine
Small Intesine
Appendix

Usually, Crohn's condition only influences locations of the large intestinal tract. Since Crohn's disease connected to the large intestinal tract, one of the most common signs is diarrhoea or irregular bowel movements, and abdominal discomfort and also cramping.

Like all autoimmune conditions, Crohn's disease is a very significant problem, and also there isn't any cure for it. There are some brand-new treatments available, but nothing that will heal it outright.

Some people appear to occasionally flare-ups from their Crohn's condition. Others deal with chronic flare their entire lives, which could sometimes cause more significant problems.

The drugs you take if you are having a flare up are immunosuppressant sorts of medications as well as steroids, neither which aren't truly all that pleasurable to swallow. They both have a lot of adverse effects, and the immunosuppressant enhance your chances of getting some opportunistic infection.

How are Emotional Stress & Crohn's Disease Linked?

Numerous people have said that forms of Inflammatory Bowel Disease, including Crohn's Disease, is caused by emotional stress, anxiety, and tension. However, this is not entirely true. While there may be related links to emotional stress and Crohn's Disease, it is not the sole reason for this disorder.

A shared misunderstanding is that Inflammatory Bowel Disease (IBD) is the same thing as Irritable Bowel Syndrome (IBS). However, these vary considerably. IBD causes inflammation of the intestines and produced psychological factors. However, there is an active link in emotional issues contributing to IBS.

Some may argue that emotion triggers Crohn's Disease, in fact, inadequate response of the immune system and no correlation to the disease and psychological issues. Nonetheless, feelings may contribute in how a person deals with Crohn's Disease.

In coping with any chronic disease, people may find difficult is dealing with the long-term effects of the medical condition. Therefore, individuals with Crohn's could become depressed or suffer other psychological issues, such as severe anxiety or dependency. As Crohn's often causes excessive diarrhoea and gas, it is sometimes embarrassing for people to go out in public, possibly leading to reclusion. Likewise, travel becomes harder, which may lead to feelings of loss of freedom. Long-term pain also causes emotional complications, as well as long-term use of pain medications.

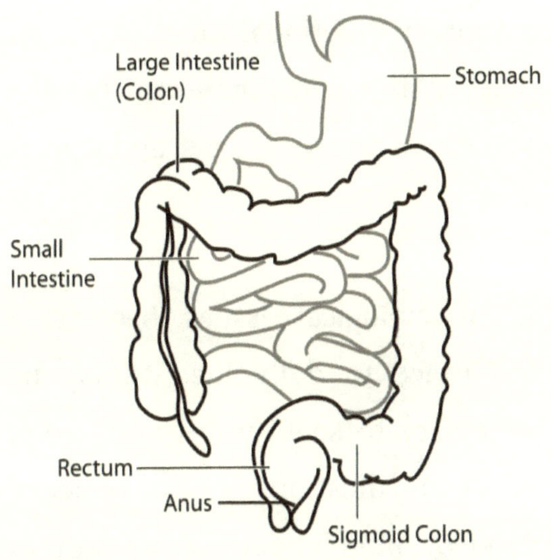

Large Intestine
(Colon)
Stomach
Small
Intestine
Rectum
Anus
Sigmoid Colon

While Crohn's Disease may cause emotional stress, there has also been a reverse connection recognised: meaning stress may cause flare-ups of complications in patients already affected by Crohn's Disease. Through extremely emotional times, a person may notice an increase in the severity of diarrhoea, gas, and pain.

If psychological issues become a hindrance to daily life, it may be necessary to seek professional help. While medication is not typically needed, merely getting support is beneficial, it might be achieved by becoming a member of a support group or speaking with other people online that may suffer from the similar or the same disorders.

There are precautions that you can need to limit stress as a result of Crohn's Disease. Keep a spare change of clothing with you and familiarise yourself with your surroundings, including the whereabouts of bathrooms, and being mindful of your reaction to particular foods, will help to ease any anxiety when you are out to eat and prepare you for any potential issues that could arise.

Food Allergic Reaction & Food Intolerance

A lot of clinical physicians nowadays are offering much focus on food allergies and intolerance unlike previously. Although no specific medicine used as a treatment for food allergic reactions, various other alternatives can be sought to regulate your addiction to particular foods. Some medical professionals additionally suggest vitamin supplements and also different other drugs that can be valuable in controlling your yearnings for sure foods.

There are good books around to read about this; about food allergic reactions, food intolerance, and treatments. It is essential to obtain vital guidance to attain durable and dramatic health and wellness improvements.

It is vital to understand how food level of sensitivities creates misdiagnosed as well as persistent conditions like migraines, constant tiredness, as well as sinus issues. By gradually identifying specific food allergies, intolerances, it can help you to improve your diet plan to achieve better health.

Some chronic ailments like the ones mentioned over remain evasive, and also physicians find it difficult to identify such illnesses. If all routine examinations cannot supply understandable medical diagnosis, the most likely wrongdoers are food intolerance and even food allergies.

You could discover clear explanations concerning the reasons, differences in between allergic reactions as well as intolerance, and also various case studies on particular problems that the readers are accustomed. Most importantly, the required services or therapies for such issues offered. Several graphs and pictures are supplied, consisting of an elimination diet plan divided into stages as well as a continuous reintroduction food system.

If you suspect that you have a persistent condition linked to any dietary sensitivity, then see your doctor.

Understanding More About Goitre

This condition affects the thyroid gland, which grows in size because o the lack or excess of essential ingredients. The thyroid gland found at the front of the throat, below the larynx known as Adam's apple. The thyroid gland plays a critical function in our system. It produces thyroid hormones known as thyroxine (T4) and triiodothyronine (T3), which goes through the body in the bloodstream. Thyroxin keeps the bodily functions in working order.

A few of the symptoms and signs which would help you detect goitre is the swelling of the throat area, which can vary in size from a tiny bump to a mass of flesh. You will face problems while swallowing your food due to expansion as well as breathing problems. As the enlarged tissue presses on to the windpipe and oesophagus, it becomes difficult to breathe and eat or swallow.

Some of the prevalent causes of goitre are:

- *Insufficient levels of iodine in the diet.*

- *Eating foods which refute the iodine in the diet.*

- *Drug intake of lithium and phenylbutazone; one of the cause is one of the reasons.*

- *The effects of thyroid cancer*

- *Nodules on the thyroid gland*

- *Hyperthyroidism (overactive thyroid gland).*

- *Hypothyroidism (underactive thyroid gland).*

There are two types of goitre classified as Endemic Goitre and Sporadic Goitre.

Endemic Goitre

It can say that this type of goitre is similar to an epidemic wherein, not an individual is affected, but the whole area or community is residing in a specific place gets changed. The lack of iodine is the primary cause, and in far-fetched situations, it becomes even more challenging to provide the proper care.

Sporadic Goitre

Here an individual is affected, and the reasons could be as common as family history, lack of iodine in the diet and women succumb to goitre more than men.

Some of the treatment options you
can try for the patients are:

- *Intake of iodine-rich diet.*

- *By using drugs as mentioned
  by your doctor, you would see
  a change in your health.*

- *Removal of the nodules
  present in the system either
  by medication or surgery.*

Leaky Gut & Multiple Sclerosis

No person recognises what causes numerous sclerosis. Throughout the globe, you will find lots of ideas on the causes of autoimmune diseases as you will identify researchers.

One relatively preferred theory states that autoimmune conditions such as bronchial asthma, multiple sclerosis, as well as Lou Gehrig's illness caused by either a form of leaking gut disorder or food level of sensitivities.

The dripping gut disorder occurs when intact, healthy proteins passed through little areas in between the intestinal walls as well as enter the bloodstream. When this happens, the immune system is turned on into assaulting these healthy proteins because to the body immune system; intact food proteins is an intruder. The problem is that these of healthy food proteins also appear like the tissue of the central nerves. When the immune system attacks the food protein, it likewise assaults the body's own myelin.

The most effective means to keep this from taking place are to first, heal the leaky gut to decrease and also with any luck avoid whole healthy food proteins from getting into the bloodstream. Moreover, 2nd quit consuming foods that contain healthy proteins that are recognised to simulate the self-proteins of the central nervous system.

Lots of people have an all-natural susceptibility to developing leaky digestive tract disorder. Points like eating food you are sensitive to, alcohol usage, infection, non-steroidal anti-inflammatory medicines, yeast overgrowth, and also parasites can trigger the little rooms in intestinal walls to obtain more significant. This will permit more food proteins to leakage right into the bloodstream.

Among the most vital points when recovering a leaking gut is exceptionally cautious concerning food level of sensitivities. People with numerous sclerosis have an allergy or ELISA test to determine which foods their body responds.

Many people with multiple sclerosis have found that by avoiding the foods, they reveal conscious by the ELISA test they have fewer flare-ups as well as a definite decrease in signs.

Candida Fungus

Candida fungus usually is inoffensive yeast, a microorganism that lives naturally inside our bodies in little populaces within the intestinal tracts. Occasionally, however, under specific problems can alter into a fungal infection. The aggressive fungal kind gets into the body's systems and creates much damage.

Exactly how does this happen and how is it dealt handled? Well, there are a variety of causes and not too many possible treatments. Before examining therapy alternatives, it is necessary to comprehend the cause of the imbalance. Usual reasons for ecological inequalities are modifications in blood sugar level levels because of diabetes mellitus, changes in hormonal agent levels as a result of pregnancy, adolescence, menopause and also menstrual cycle. Modifications in typical gut vegetations because of intestinal tract infections or the intake of antibiotics, or a jeopardised immune system, such as AIDS.

The fungal type of Candida is a much worse companion compared to the pure yeast infection. The fungal-form of Candida creates aggressive origins that penetrate the intestinal walls, as well as create the possibility for partially digested food fragments to pass through the bloodstream, and develop food sensitivities. The fungus additionally ferments the sugars in our colon. This could cause an issue with gas, excessive bloating of the belly, and also extreme discomfort.

The fungal type of Candida likewise assaults the nervous system. Victims of fungal Candida experience mood swings, anxiety, fogginess of the mind, as well as reduced focus. There are several concepts regarding why this occurs. They are just that, concepts. One such idea is that when the fungus pierces the wall of the intestinal tract and enables the partially digested food to pass into the bloodstream, exorphins are released. They could influence the neurological responses by switching them on and off. Thus producing the anxiety as well as mood swings.

There are hormone changes associated with fungal Candida. Severe menstruation pain, thyroid conditions, as well as auto-immune deficiencies are known to be an outcome of fungal Candida. Various other symptoms that are hormone related and indicate a Candida overgrowth are discomfort in the muscle mass and also joints, sugar yearnings, professional athlete's foot, yeast infection of the mouth, sinusitis, poor concentration, and even intolerance of perfume.

There are diets and treatments available to clear your body of this terrible fungus, but they typically aren't quick fixes, as well as often the damages to your body's body organs can be permanent. A number of the even more natural treatments are cranberry remove as well as garlic. Various other products to be dealt with once you have begun to free your body of the fungal infection are the leaking gut and also general detoxification, since Candida could generate as much as 100 different toxins.

Cancer & Spicy Foods

Spicy Foods

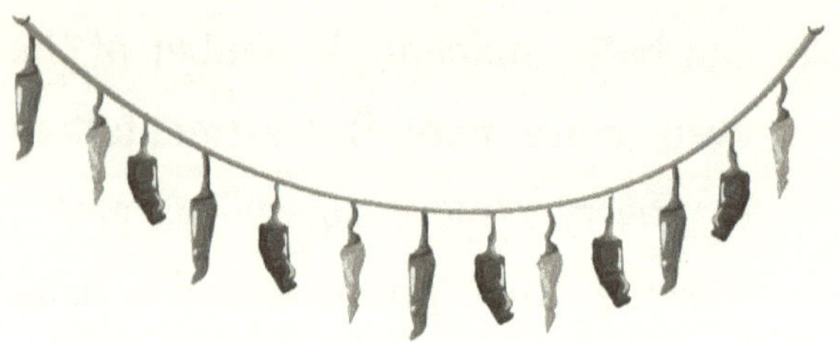

Spicy foods containing peppers might have an impact on disease. According to research capsaicin, found in hot peppers like jalapeno, habanero, and chilli destroyed prostate cancer cells. Furthermore, it substantially decreased the development of prostate cancer in rats. Hot peppers contain antioxidants which help neutralise free radicals, potentially harmful substances because of lifestyle and metabolic factors. Garlic used in spicy food has a positive impact on cancer, as a preventative and an immune booster that encourages your body to fight any cancer cells.

Hot peppers might increase stomach acidity, increase the risk of bleeding from blood-thinning medications and decrease the effectiveness of aspirin. Consult your doctor about consuming spicy food if you have a stomach or intestinal problem, or are taking blood-thinning medications or aspirin

Mushrooms

Studies have found that mushrooms might enable white blood cells to act aggressively against foreign bacteria. The best types of mushrooms are maitake and shiitake.

In this last section, we have looked at various autoimmune diseases and how you can help yourself, the importance of what genetics, lifestyle and you eat. Let us look at ways this can be improved.

Improving Immunity & Inflammatory Conditions

More Tips for Boosting the Body's Immune System

Millions of microorganisms are continuously attacking the human body; this is why it is important not to take your immune system for granted.

What can you do to help keep your immune system healthy and ready to shield your body from infection? To answer this question, Shaklee Corporation recently formed the Centre for Immune Research, which offers these valuable guidelines:

Relax

Stress produces many effects on the endocrine systems; scientists believe that chronic stresses may diminish immune function. There are some techniques to help you relax, such as deep breathing or yoga, which can reduce mental and physical pressure or stress as well as lower blood pressure and slow down your heart rate.

Sleep

Not getting enough sleep leaves you feeling irritable, less focused, forgetful, sluggish which can temporarily limit the activity of particular cells in the immune system to work, by up to 50 percent.

Ensure you get seven to eight hours sleep each night.

Sleep deprivation can cause:

- *Irritability*
- *Cognitive impairment*
- Impaired Immune System
- *Memory lapses or loss*
- *Impaired judgment*
- *Severe yawning*
- *Hallucinations*
- *Symptoms similar to ADHD*
- *Risk of diabetes Type 2*
- *Increased heart rate variability*
- *Risk of heart disease*
- *Increased reaction time*
- *Decreased accuracy*
- *Tremors and aches*

- *Growth suppression*
- *Risk of obesity*

Feed your immune system

Not enough calories and too much dietary fat can weaken the immune response. Nutritionists endorse a well-balanced diet that includes lots of fruit, vegetables, low-fat dairy products and whole grains.

Physical Activity and Exercise

Daily exercise helps strengthen the immune system, cardiovascular system, bones, heart, and muscles. It also stimulates the release of endorphins, and improves our concentration and mental functioning, as well as lowering cholesterol levels and blood pressure; possibly reducing cortisol and other stress hormones as well.

Learn about interferon

Most people have not heard of interferon, which is a natural protein that helps to protect the body from daily exposure to germs, which can often lead to severe infections. When an invading virus assaults a cell, interferon then notifies nearby cells to take action and then triggers their cell resistance mechanisms. Interferon can activate other immune cells that destroy invading pathogens.

Due to interferon playing a crucial part in immune system health, the Shaklee Corporation has been raising awareness about NutriFeron which is a new dietary supplement, which naturally escalates the body's production of its interferon. Initially, a Japanese scientist discovered interferon at Tokyo University.

After more than forty years of research, he developed NutriFeron on natural interferon-inducing compounds. Medical professionals and scientists have explored NutriFeron as a blended formula of plant extracts that naturally lifts levels of interferon, and assists the immune at a cellular level (see www.shaklee.com), check with a medical doctor before taking this.

The Amazing Health Benefits of Pure Water

We ought to pay attention to the amount of water we drink; it is so important because it affects our health. However, what is pure water? It does not tap water. Pure water is a very high-quality bottled spring water, or water filtered through a high-quality water filter.

It is crucial that your water is pure water because tap water has so many contaminations and impurities that it is harmful to your health. The main issue with tap water is the chemicals used to purify water from pathogens. The majority of water sources use chemicals like chlorine, and other compounds that are unhealthy, and tap water initially comes from low-quality sources, for example, the big city. They often obtain their water from the local river that is not clean. Many upstream towns discarded (treated) sewage into these rivers. Also, many farms upstream have contributed agricultural chemicals into this poisons mix. Most individuals would not even eat any fish caught in the river, where the drinking water had come.

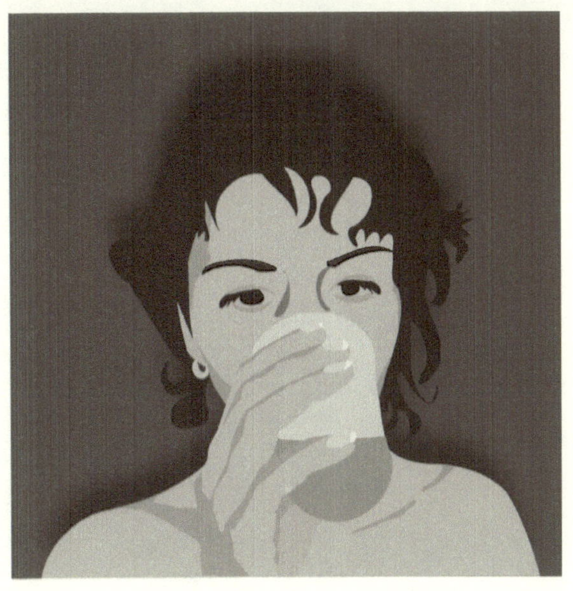

So, when you have pure drinking water - what are the health benefits of drinking plenty of water?

Your body consists of mostly water,
and when you drink a lot of it, your
body functions better.

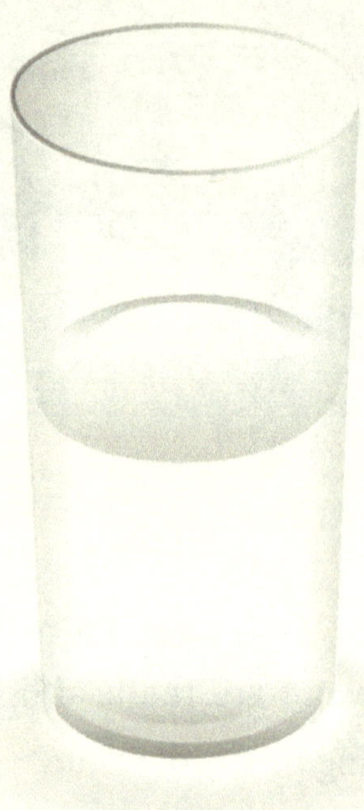

Weight Loss

Research has found that those who drink plenty of water are more inclined to lose weight in comparison to individuals who do not drink enough or any water at all. The reason for this is because the water removes the toxins stored in the body fat. Otherwise, the body cannot burn fat.

Removal of Toxins

After the body takes in toxins every day which includes food you eat, the water you drink and the air you breathe, are full of toxins. A right amount of pure water every day all day flushes out the body, and it removes the toxins from your body such as the liver, joints, fat, and other places the toxins stored.

Improved Intestinal Health

Drinking plenty of water helps the digestive system to function better; the majority of issues associated with the gastrointestinal tract.

Other Benefits

Water is the essential nutrient that the body requires. When you drink much water, and I mean plenty; every system in the body, the organs to cells, benefits. Of course, it helps if it is pure water. Start drinking plenty of pure water every day and observe how the benefits increase.

Have you considered what the result would be if you drink water as your primary liquid drink? Ailments such as excess body fat, skin disorders, stomach pains, heart issues, and other health issues may result from drinking consuming sugary fizzy drinks. The best replacement drink is water.

1. Lose Weight

You can lose weight quickly. If you quit trying to lose weight on a strict diet, just replacing your intake with water, can help you to reduce your weight.

2. Boost Metabolism

Boost your metabolism, research studies have shown that drinking less than 20 fluid ounces of water in the morning, increases metabolism. Should you not drink water daily at a specific time, perhaps place a reminder in your calendar or mobile phone. In no time will you feel the difference in your energy levels and also body weight.

3. Improve Brain Function

Your brain will improve. Our brains consist of 75%+ water right? Thus, drinking water makes total sense for boosting your mental function. Drinking water enables you to focus and keep up mental energy for psychological tasks.

4. Prevents Overeating

Drinking more water this prevents you from overeating, and you will not require expensive pills and appetite suppressants. The amount of water you drink signals your brain that you are full and so you consume fewer calories.

5. Eliminate Toxins and Waste Faster

It eliminates waste and toxins by detoxifying your body on a daily basis; toxins build up and can cause health problems.

Consuming plenty of water daily is most important if you do have cancer. Numerous signs and symptoms that cancer patients experience, for example, exhaustion or queasiness, are honestly related to dehydration, including blood clotting due to the drugs taken during treatment. Radiation treatment treatments can often increase your need for water because the medications are tough on your liver.

Added fluids help to protect your liver from further damage. On the other hand, significant dehydration can even cause cancer in the body if poisonous toxins not flushed out of the body.

6. Less Risk of Disease

You decrease the risk of encouraging diseases such as diabetes, liver disease, hypertension, and heart problems. Related problems have a higher risk of developing when you do not drink enough water so drink enough to help prevent them.

7. Clear Skin

Your skin will be clear and smoother. We all need to try things from the inside out to see real results in our appearance. Water will help moisturise and clear -up any skin disorders from the inside out, so you do not have to pile on skincare products.

8. Save Money

Lastly, it will save you money because it is cheaper than buying fizzy drinks. Plus your health and purse will thank you.

In summary, beware of sensationalistic claims about the type of perfect diet to follow because there is determined by many other factors including where individuals live, cultural and environmental factors, etc.

The most common advice is to eat a balanced diet, drink plenty of water, eat plenty of vegetables and fruits; try and avoid processed foods and extreme eating habits such as under-eating and over-eating.

The majority of individuals believe the digestive system is a location whereby food is broken down, and nutrients transported throughout the body. However, fewer people are aware that the digestive system's associated with the immune system.

The digestive system is about just under 90% of the immune system.

Bad bacteria feed on sugars; those living in civilised countries frequently experience health issues related to a lack of probiotics in their system.

This lack of probiotics is directly related to our diet and is the result of excess:

- *Agricultural chemicals and pesticides*
- *Chlorinated water*
- *Processed foods*
- *Pollution*
- *Probiotic Supplements Curb Sugar Cravings*
- *Sugar Artificial sweeteners*

Research has concluded that consuming probiotics have a much better positive influence on our immune system and general health than a daily multivitamin. Furthermore, studies have found that using a probiotic supplement results in significant loss of weight, in comparison to non-probiotic taking individuals.

Any weight loss in connection with probiotic supplements appears to be a direct result of probiotics capability to curb sugar cravings. The limited need for sugar starves off dangerous parasites, bacteria, and yeast that feed in the presence of sugar.

Probiotic supplements have shown a significant decrease in sugar cravings in a few days; this destroys harmful microorganisms and gives you consistent energy.

Excessive sugar cravings may be a sign of probiotic deficiency. Deal with this deficiency by supplementing your diet with a high-quality probiotic supplement.

Encouraging your specific body food may help keep your insusceptible framework stable. In case you are searching for approaches to counteract winter colds and this season's cold virus. Plan your dinner with these immune system booster foods and can strengthen your immune system.

Organic Citrus Fruits

Many people swing to vitamin C after they have gotten a bug. That is because it helps to strengthen your immune system. Vitamin C is thought to build the generation of white platelets. These are vital for battling contamination.

The main citrus products you can have are:

- *Grapefruit*
- *Oranges*
- *Tangerines*
- *Lemons*

Since your body does not deliver or store it, you require day to day vitamin C for wellbeing. All organic citrus products are high in vitamin

Citrus fruits like oranges, lemons, limes, tangerines, grapefruits are a rich source of Vitamin C. Vitamin C plays a vital role in encouraging the immune system; resisting microorganisms entering the body by boosting white cell production that helps fight against infections.

Ways to Make Use of Citrus Juices to Ease Constipation

Citrus Juices

Citrus juices are an irregular bowel movements treatment that is a superb method to boost your colon and other parts of the body. Given that your colon is less energetic during the night drinking juices as quickly as you stir up and also rise could promote stable peristaltic activity and also promote a bowel movement.

Lemons

Lemons are full of minerals, especially potassium, Vitamin C, and bioflavonoids. They have a cleaning activity for the entire body.

Fresh lemon juice contains citric acid, which acts in the body in such a way nothing else juice does. Initially, it acts upon the liver to build up its enzymes so it can detoxify toxic substances in the blood. Then it integrates with calcium to form soluble chemical substances. This makes it reliable in getting rid of kidney and also pancreatic stones, plaque can develop along artery wall surfaces and various other calcium deposits that occur in the body.

When the liver, gallbladder, as well as pancreas, are not functioning well food digestion is affected. This can develop into bowel irregularity.

Use lemons reasonably considering that they separate oils throughout food digestion and in our body, they make oils much less available to our cells as well as joints.

If you have lemon allergies or ulcers after that, you should prevent lemon juice. If you have arthritis lemons are not a great selection.

1. Press one lemon into a glass of distilled water. Consume it first thing when you get up. Don't consume alcohol or anything else for a minimum of 1/2 hr.

2. You could utilise a citrus press to juice the lemon or squeeze it to get the juice out.

Grapefruit Juice

Another constipation treatment you could utilise is consuming alcohol a glass of fresh squeezed grapefruit first thing in the early morning. Once again wait a minimum of 1/2 hour before you eat anything.

Grapefruit and Orange Juice

Drink a combination of grapefruit and orange juice first thing in the morning.

Warning

Please note that if you are taking any anticonvulsant medications, contraceptive pill, estrogen, protease preventions or various other sorts of medicines avoid alcohol consumption and grapefruit juice. It slows down the malfunction of specific drugs allowing them to increase in the blood to dangerous levels.

Avocados

Avocados are rich in potassium and vitamin A besides containing folic acid and magnesium.

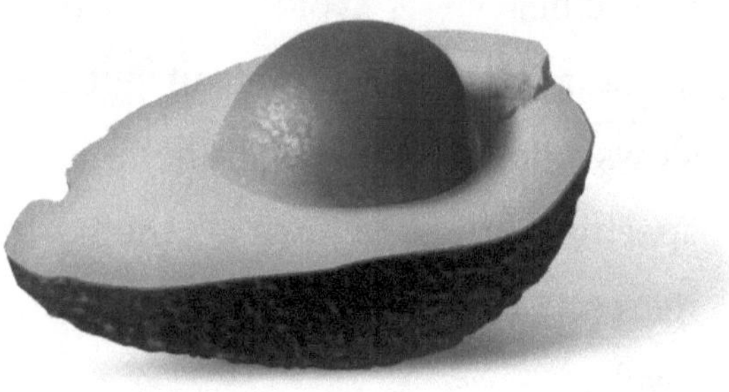

Broccoli

Broccoli is supercharged with vitamins and minerals. Pressed with vitamins A, C, and E, and also numerous different cell reinforcements and fibre.

Broccoli is supercharged with vitamins A, C, and E, minerals, antioxidants, and fibre that protect your body from damage. A daily serving of broccoli soup can work wonders in boosting your immune system.

To make soup, boil broccoli in chicken or vegetable stock and add it to a mixture of garlic, shallots, leeks, onion, and thyme cooked in butter.

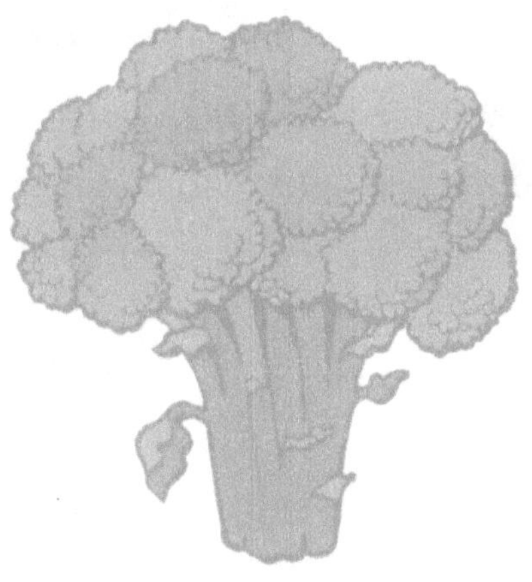

Vegetables such as broccoli, Brussel sprouts, cabbage, and cauliflower, are excellent sources of beta-carotene and help protect against free-radical damage. They also contain vitamin C and calcium.

Button Mushrooms

Button mushrooms are a rich source of Selenium; types of Vitamin B complex such as Niacin and Riboflavin, that are known to be proven ways for preventing colds and flu and there have been some unconfirmed information suggesting it is useful in avoiding tumours too.

The dark-coloured fruit is regarded as the superfood and is rich in the super antioxidant, Anthocyanins.

Some data have suggested that Acai berries are among the right options to boost the immunity when it degenerates with age.

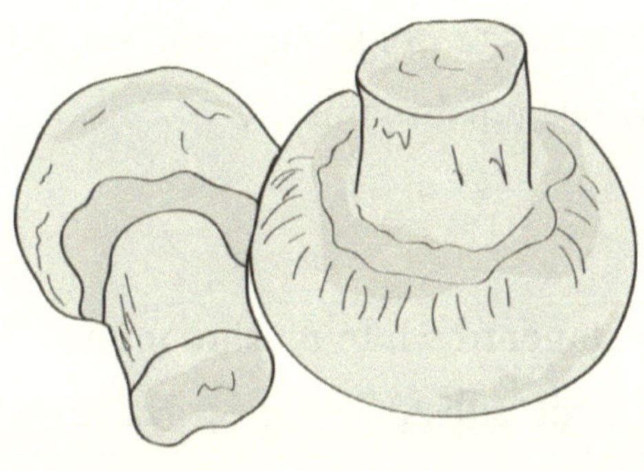

Avoid eating mushrooms raw although it is highly unlikely that you will get cancer from eating a few white mushrooms alone. However, the combination of the other toxins we eat or exposed to, it is best not to risk eating them uncooked.

It is advisable always to cook edible white mushrooms (Agaricus bisporus) because raw mushrooms can be toxic.

The main reasons why you should cook raw mushrooms:

The standard white mushroom has a few toxic substances, i.e., agaritine. Agartine has been found to be carcinogenic in mice, and is, therefore, a suspected carcinogen for humans. Recent studies indicate that the risk for humans is low.

In the liver, agaritine is broken down into glutamic acid, and the hydrazine is responsible for the carcinogenic properties of agaritine. As agaritine is not heat-stable, heating mushrooms boiled or fried further reduces any potential risk.

The second reason is to heat the mushrooms to kill any potential pathogenic bacteria; mushrooms cultivated on horse manure. The manure sterilised before use, but it is still a viable medium for bacterial growth. There is thus a considerable risk for pathogenic bacteria to be present on raw mushrooms. Cooking (or frying) destroys the bacteria (including the potential pathogens) on the surface of the mushroom

Chinese cabbage

Chinese cabbage– is an excellent source of vitamin A.

Elderberry

An old and classic remedy for the treatment and prevention of flu. Elderberries have the presence of Antioxidants which prevent free radicals from destroying the cell membranes. This action also helps in preventing the oxidative stress.

Garlic

Garlic is a common ingredient these days because it adds flavour to cooking and an absolute necessity for your wellbeing. Garlic's insusceptible boosting properties appear to originate from a substantial grouping of sulfur-containing mixes, antibacterial, antiviral and antifungal. These properties increase immune function. It is a good source of selenium; a vital trace element, and sulfur, which is essential for healthy liver function.

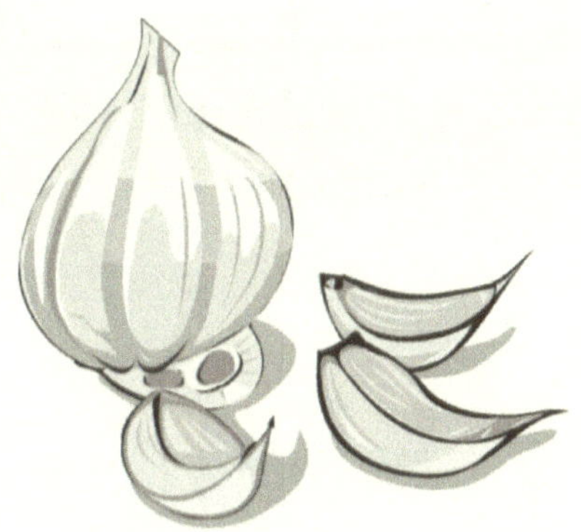

Ginger

Ginger is another best remedy for fixing many problems in the wake of becoming ill. Ginger encourages the body to fend off infection and traditionally used in treating colds and flu.

Ginger may help diminish irritation, which can help lessen a sore throat and other provocative diseases. While utilised as a part of many sweet pastries, ginger packs some warmth as gingerol. Ginger may help diminish perpetual torment and may have cholesterol-bringing down properties.

Green tea

Both green and dark teas pressed with flavonoids, a kind of cell reinforcement. Green tea contains amino corrosive L-theanine that helps in the generation of germ-battling mixes in your T-cells.

Horseradish

Horseradish contains oils that have demonstrated antibiotic properties, and have been effective against infections.

Kiwi

Kiwis contain various supplements, including folate, potassium, vitamin K, and vitamin C. Vitamin C supports white platelets to battle contamination, while kiwi's different supplements keep your body working legitimately.

Kiwifruit, blueberries, and oranges are all excellent sources of vitamin C. To increase the amount of vitamin C from your oranges; you can thinly peel the skin off with a knife, leaving the white bioflavonoid rich inner peel.

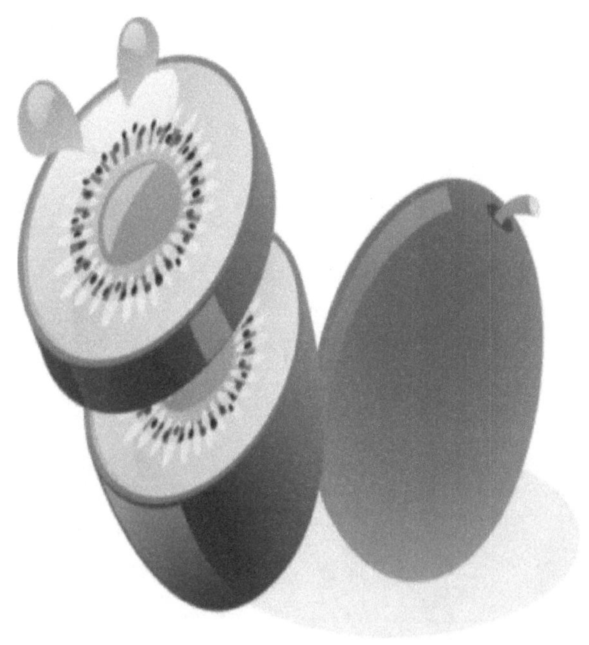

Leek and Onions

Leeks and onions are an excellent source of sulfur and contain the similar properties as garlic.

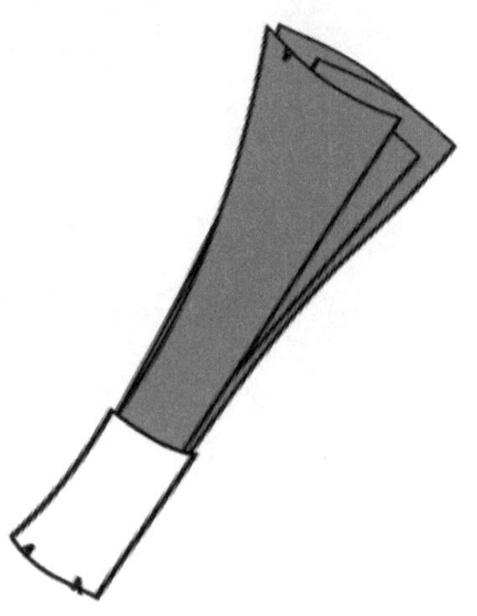

Health Advantages of Onions

There are plenty of wellness benefits from onions so if you enjoy them to snack on or to prepare with don't hesitate to proceed to do so. There are various kinds of antioxidants found in onions that can assist to enhance your body immune system. Some research has revealed they also help to combat versus diabetic issues, cardiovascular disease, as well as some sorts of cancers. Onions contain significant quantities of chromium as well as Vitamin C that your body needs as well.

In current research studies, people with high blood pressure and high cholesterol levels actually could substantially reduce those numbers. All they did was include onions in their diet daily for thirty days. Of course, there is some conflict regarding the legitimacy of such test outcomes. It is because of some people making other changes too that could represent their blood pressure and cholesterol dropping.

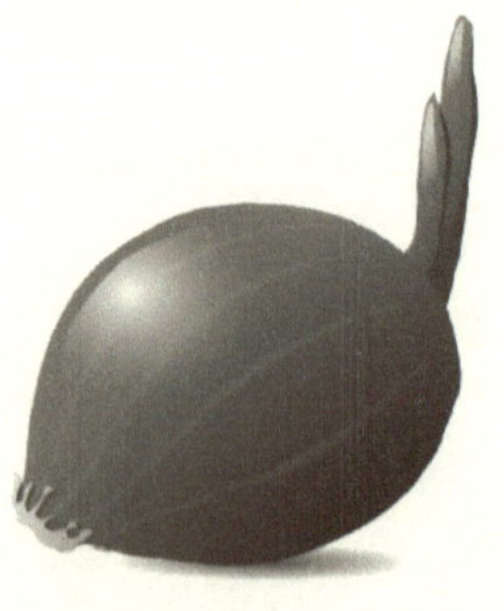

Onions are beneficial and help osteoporosis or those not getting enough calcium as they grow older. Moreover, tests reveal that consuming onions could help to balance out the impact of osteoporosis.

In some cultures, onions are a staple in a sort of brew offered to those that have dealt with malnutrition; given to those that are in the procedure of recouping from serious illnesses or broken bones. They think there are properties in onions that will assist to promote the recovery process.

In the early days, onions given to individuals with colds, bronchitis, or even asthma. Lots of people still count on these natural home remedies, and also they use them instead of getting over the counter drugs or prescription medicines. It may sound strange to some individuals, but for those that have had advantages, this is the only technique used.

There are different health and wellness benefits of onions, but research has yet to fully verified this; more research needs to validate or reject such claims. However, precisely what is known is that onion is a vegetable that is both tasty and also benefits you. For that reason, you need to enjoy consuming it too.

Orange Vegetables

Sweet potatoes, carrots, pumpkin, and squash are an excellent source of vitamin A.

Oysters

They are rich in the wound healing Zinc and are believed to be vital for male fertility as well.

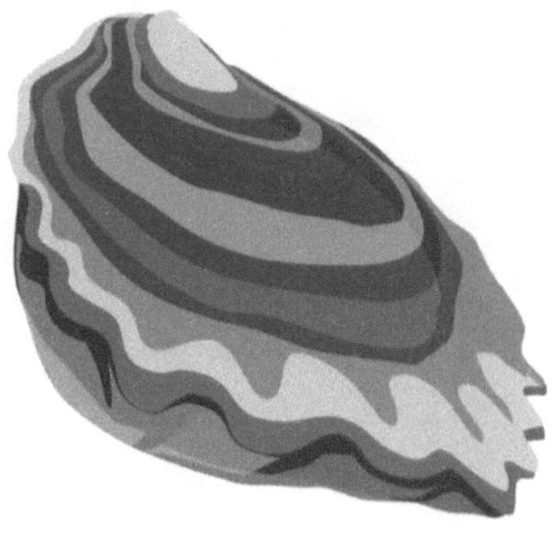

Red Bell peppers

If you think organic citrus products have the most vitamin C of any natural product or vegetable, rethink once. Ounce for ounce, red bell peppers contain twice as much vitamin C as citrus. They are adding a rich wellspring of beta-carotene. Other than boosting your resistance power, vitamin C may help keep up the healthy skin. Beta-carotene keeps your eyes and skin stable.

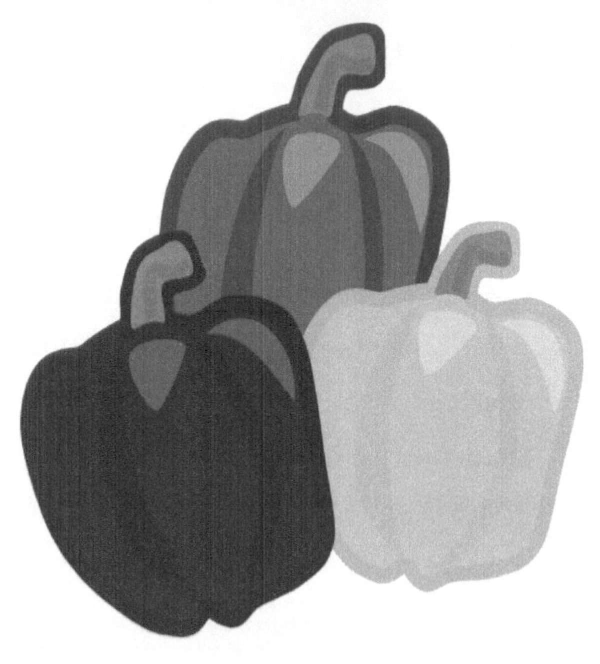

Spinach

Spinach made our rundown, not because it is rich in vitamin C, packed with various cancer prevention agents and beta-carotene, which may build the disease-battling capacity of our invulnerable frameworks. Like broccoli, spinach is most beneficial when it is cooked as meagre as conceivable with the goal that it holds its supplements.

Spinach and other leafy greens contain beta-carotene, the precursor to vitamin A, vitamin C, and calcium.

Turmeric

You may know turmeric supplements are essential fixing in many ways. In any case, this splendid yellow, astringent zest has likewise utilised for a considerable length of time as a calming in treating both osteoarthritis and joint pain. Turmeric enhances the immune system and has a detoxifying effect.

Water Melon

Glutathione is the immune enhancing nutrient in the watermelon, which helps in boosting the natural defence of the body against diseases. The water content and refreshing abilities of watermelon have also added beneficial effects on the human body.

Healthy or Physically Fit

To build and develop a happy, productive life means that you keep yourself healthy not physically but emotionally, and spiritually too. Research studies have shown that those who go to church, volunteer, or belong to a club are often more able to experience much better health than those who do not interact in social activities, on a regular basis.

A holistic health outlook is not only achieved just by exercising, eating the right things, and sleeping well. These factors are essential in enabling us to live a healthier life. Countless people have used prayer or spiritual healing, especially when becoming ill. Those facing illness most often turn to religion for their strength and help. Most people believe that by having strong faith, it can help them to recover from illness and maintain good health.

Mind, body, and soul takes care of us not spiritually but physically also. It is crucial in the way we take care of ourselves. When you take care of yourself physically, you will begin to notice an escalation in energy levels. Before this, you may be lacking in energy, feeling fatigue; feeling sleepy. When you started to focus on health and began to take better care of yourself, you will feel more emotionally stable and spiritually aware and in touch with yourself; understanding yourself far better in the process.

Imagine physically, looking a new person, and spiritually feeling like a new person. Your self -esteem will rise immensely. So, by experiencing and looking healthy, you will begin to see yourself as a desirable person whom you can be proud. Once you start to feel very proud of yourself, you will start to feel like no job is too high or hard for you to achieve.

Jane in her early forties began to realise the importance of taking care of herself. Years ago, she went to see the doctor because she was feeling sluggish and fatigue. Her doctor thought Jane was extremely overweight for my age, build, and height. She was forty-two, five foot two and 148 pounds. The doctor said if Jane lost weight, she would feel far better about herself both physically and mentally. By losing the weight, she would help overcome her fatigue and help herself emotionally, physically and spiritually. Personally, Jane was feeling down and unhappy with my physical appearance. She realised that she could no longer let herself become any heavier.

The first thing Jane did to help herself get physically back into shape was changing her lifestyle and her eating habits. If she were going to lose any weight, and get back into shape, she had to change the way she consumed food. Jane loved to eat good food, just like most individuals. She had an appetite particularly for fatty foods, candy, cream cheese and other healthful foods that are not that good for our bodies.

The message here is to pay attention to what you are eating and eliminate unhealthy foods that are not compatible with your metabolism. Most people's metabolism is different, so eat healthy foods that work best for you. For example, Jane's body reacted well to carbohydrates whereas her husband's body retains mostly water if he ingests many carbs into his system.

Jane began eating mainly proteins and eliminated most fatty foods as best she could. We require the right fats in our meal plan, but make sure they are the right types of fats. Be aware of those fat-free foods they have in the supermarkets. They say they have zero fat, yet the calories are as bad as a fatty food, with many fat grams in it. To make the fat-free foods taste good, they use plenty of sugar, which then causes you to gain weight. It does not make sense.

An If you feel your weight is okay, then carry on eating healthy, to keep in shape and to maintain your weight. Most of what you eat affects you. Try to even out the number of calories you eat day after you have decided on the number of calories you will eat and cut down where you can.

You can stop eating full-fat cheeses unless they are fat-free. Jane eliminated bread and food products that were very high-fat content. When it absorbed into your body, it transforms into sugar and appears to increase the appetite. Soon, you will be hungry again, and you want to eat more.

Delicious Chinese food can be high in carbohydrates, and I notice this seems to have the same effect. However, the calories keep mounting up, and the salt content in Chinese food certainly makes me feel incredibly bloated, and thirsty.

Perhaps read the food content labels when you shop in the supermarket. I have eaten a lot of fat-free foods, low in calories. I looked at the product that I was buying had less sodium and sugar in it. It is the first step in getting back on track. Also, eat fewer fat grams as possible each day.

We hear this regularly, but drinking water is so important to eat healthily.

Jane made sure she drank plenty of water as much as her body could hold, which is also essential. If you are getting your body in shape, and lose weight water, this often helps to flush away unwanted impurities and toxins from your system.

The body contains around 50% to 70% water. Because the water cannot remain indefinitely stored in the body, we need to replace it frequently. As you know, water contains zero fat grams or calories, and so it is one of the healthiest drinks to indulge in very often, throughout the day. Adults need to consume at least two to three litres of liquid daily. I know it sounds a lot, but you are going to the bathroom, perspiring, etc. and so you lose the fluids you drink too.

When Jane became hungry during the day, she made sure she snacked on healthy foods like yoghurt and bananas. She also eliminated unhealthy foods, like ice cream, potato chips or crisps, sugary cakes, etc. Jane would eat meats such as turkey or chicken. Meats do contain valuable nutrients like protein. However, be careful because some meat contains cholesterol also.

Try to leave out the salad cream or mayonnaise, tomato ketchup, and the foods that easily add to putting on the weight, and also hold water.

It does help if you try to eat slowly. Because eating slowly, you enjoy your meal more, and not eat as much. Eating your lunch, for example, should take around 20 minutes not 5 minutes!

Jane also made sure she ate her breakfast first thing in the morning. She noticed that when she had no breakfast, Jane would go on to eat more and more during the day; grazing was the term Jane had convinced herself of or, she ate later on at dinnertime.

You need to avoid eating huge dinners because the food then lies in your stomach all evening, and you will not burn many calories; the food stays in your stomach. Jane's regular diet was a healthy breakfast, snack, lunch and dinner, and later, a light meal. She felt fulfilled and did lose thirty-five pounds over time, which is a healthier way.

Losing so much weight helped Jane because she then was able to decrease her medication dosage she had been taking after she consulted with her doctor. After she began to lose the weight, her appetite declined, and she felt far better physically and emotionally. Jane felt better, and her inner self-began to blossom, she felt content and happy again.

In this last section, we covered the benefits of all kinds of natural organic foods. It is fascinating to research some of the benefits of natural foods we so often take for granted. By making healthy and straightforward adjustments, it is possible to maintain a robust immune system and lose weight, if that is your intention too.

Next, let us now look at the last section and the importance of nutrition.

Nutrition &
Eating for Health

The Importance of Nutrition

The roadway to a healthy and balanced way of life is through the proper amount of nutrition. An inequality of such may trigger poor health, fatigue and also a weakened immune system. To have the healthy nutrients needed to maintain health, people have to have amino acids, vitamins, fats, sugars, etc. Along with everyday wellness, nutrition plays a significant role in sports performance. The factor is because the appropriate amount of food enhances strength, energy, and ability.

Some professionals believe that nourishment might additionally be related to long life. Sound judgment informs us that the healthier we are, the stronger our body immune system ends up being as well as, the less most likely we are to get specific illnesses. However, the sound judgment does not mean that the chance of certain diseases eliminated. However, our bodies might be better able to fight against them with the proper amount of nutrition and also a healthy and balanced immune system.

Individuals could discover nutritional components by reading the outdoors packaging of any food before they acquire it. Many individuals read labels to learn more about a food's nutritional value and whether it will be an appropriate component of their current diet regimen. Others, who are not on a diet, like to read nourishment tags to thoroughly view what they consume in hopes of keeping a healthy and balanced lifestyle.

Just as it is imperative to have nutrition in our lives, it is as essential that we not take in too much of any one nutrient. As the adage suggests, "too much of a great thing is bad." An excess amount of specific nutrients, just as a shortage of the very same, can produce hormonal variations. Also, particular vitamins can be hazardous if consumed in large quantities. The very best method to make sure that you are obtaining the right amount of nourishment in your diet plan is to talk to a specialist, who could analyse your existing medical problem as well as advise a means to increase your body immune system without harming it while doing so.

It is essential to research into nutrition is undertaken as a healthy way of living and how the absence thereof could lead to significant health problems, including psychological conditions, certain kinds of cancer and various other ill results.

Remember all the information in this book are for educational purposes only, and should not be used instead of, professional medical advice. Anyone with questions surrounding their nutritional intake or need tips on a well-balanced diet is, needs to check out an accredited dietician for additional details as well as referrals.

Nutritional Secrets Untold

A mutual understanding of nourishment and how you can make use of the information will be incredibly satisfying for anybody. We could all protect ourselves against disease and fight infection utilising an effective medicine 'Food'. Using nutrition, and supplementing your diet regimen is the vital to fat loss as well as muscle gain. Have a look at these Nutritional Secrets as well as find how to remain disease free, really feel great and look fantastic.

How Much Is Protein Needed?

Protein is a typical part of our diet regimen; a nutrient commonly distributed amongst pet and plant foods, and also it plays several essential functions in the body. Nutritional protein has two possible fates; it can be either utilised in growth as well as repair work or shed for power, like carb and also fat.

Why Carbohydrates?

Carbohydrates supply power to out the body, fibre discovered in *grains, potatoes, fruits,* as well as vegetables.

Over the last few years, research into food and blood glucose reaction has transformed our carb category system. Its found that it is difficult to predict the effect on blood glucose levels in certain foods. Instead, individuals fed carbohydrate foods and the feedback gauged. This feedback is known as the Glycemic Index (GI), it is a measure of precisely how swiftly carbohydrate foods are absorbed and taken in, as shown by elevated blood sugar. The slower the rate of blood glucose raises the reduced the GI.

Super Foods

In the food industry, super-foods are called "practical foods." These foods offer a health advantage beyond the original provision of nutrients or power and typically target a specific condition or condition.

What Super-Foods Provide

Vitamins and Minerals

An appropriate consumption of vitamin and minerals attained with a balanced diet regimen. However, there might be the reasoning for supplements in specific nutrients.

Herbals

The newest natural ones include Echinacea, gingko, and St John's Wart. They do not pitch themselves as lifesavers. However, a lot more like life-maximises, assisting you to get through the day with less interruption from colds, memory failings, mood swings, and much more.

Supplements

To supplement or otherwise to enhance, that is the question. There are different reasons that individuals might be interested in supplements. One is the issue concerning obtaining appropriate nutrients from our food supply. There is, however a suspicion that pharmaceuticals and diet plans alone, will not achieve optimal nutrition.

Nevertheless, consumers can spend large amounts of money on items that have little or no tried and tested efficiency. It is a huge money-making industry.

The Bottom Line On Supplements

Your diet may accomplish your objectives, but select only products that show the number of active ingredients on the label. Know that "all-natural" does not mean 'secure'; some natural supplements could have unpleasant adverse effects. Do not treat severe clinical conditions yourself. Go over supplement use with your doctor. If you are expectant mother or breastfeedding, seek advice from a physician before taking supplements.

Eat the Good Fats

Eat the right fats, feel and look fantastic; Authorities currently agree that fat is necessary for preserving optimum wellness. If great healthy and balanced skin, as well as rapid metabolic process, are what you want then you need to eat some fat. The great fats found in fish, nuts, and also seeds, avocados, and even cold pushed oils. Stay clear of deep-fried foods and hydrogenated fats as these raising cholesterol and clog arteries.

Consume A Variety Of Foods

For protection from most of the diseases such as cardiovascular disease and cancer cells, you need a selection of foods that provide that mix of nutrients and minerals. The goal is to eat various coloured vegetables and fruits.

Try to consume a different food each month. Eat an apple a day as the apple pectin cleans the body's gastrointestinal system by removing contaminants as well as a result of protecting against degenerative health problems such as cancer.

In conclusion, everything we eat plays a vital role in our well being and balance is essential. If you could implement just a few of these tips into your everyday routine, I am confident that you will undoubtedly

see the benefits in the not too distant
future.

Fruits & Vegetables

Fruit and vegetables are packed with nutrients, called antioxidants, that are very good for you. You can eat more fruits and vegetables of any kind to your diet. Eating ore of this helps your health, and some foods will be higher in antioxidants than others.

The three major antioxidant vitamins are:

- *beta-carotene*
- *vitamin C*
- *vitamin E.*

You will discover them in colourful fruits and vegetables, particularly those with purple, red, blue, yellow and orange.

Beta-carotene and other carotenoids:

- *Apricots*
- *Asparagus*
- *Beets*
- *Broccoli*
- *Cantaloupe*
- *Carrots*
- *Collard greens*
- *Corn*
- *Green peppers*
- *Kale*
- *Mangoes*
- *Nectarines,*

- *Peaches*
- *Pink grapefruit*
- *Pumpkin*
- *Squash*
- *Spinach*
- *Sweet potato*
- *Tangerines*
- *Tomatoes*
- *Turnip*
- *Watermelon*

Vitamin C:

- *Bell peppers*
- *Berries*
- *Broccoli*
- *Brussels sprouts*
- *Cantaloupe*
- *Cauliflower*
- *Grapefruit*
- *Honeydew*
- *Kale*
- *Kiwi*
- *Mango*
- *Nectarine*
- *Orange*
- *Papaya*
- *Snow peas*
- *Sweet potato*
- *Strawberries*
- *Tomatoes*

Vitamin E:

- *Broccoli*
- *Avocado*
- *Chard*
- *Mustard*
- *Turnip greens*
- *Mangoes*
- *Nuts*
- *Papaya*
- *Pumpkin*
- *Red peppers*
- *Spinach*
- *Sunflower seeds*

Rich in antioxidants:

- *Alfalfa sprouts*
- *Apples*
- *Beans*
- *Eggplant*
- *Plums*
- *Prunes*
- *Raisins*
- *Red grapes*
- *Onions*

Other antioxidants include:

- *Zinc*
- *Oysters*
- *Red meat*
- *Poultry*
- *Beans*
- *Nuts*
- *Seafood*
- *Whole grains*
- *Certain fortified cereals (check the ingredients if zinc been added)*
- *Dairy products*

Selenium:

- *Brazil nuts*
- *Tuna*
- *Beef*
- *Poultry*
- *Fortified bread*
- *Other grain products*

The most significant benefits of antioxidants are to eat most of these foods either raw or lightly steamed. Never overcook them.

Conclusion

In conclusion, everything we eat is vital to our well being and balance is most essential. So before you embark on the next fad diet, take a closer look what it might do to your body.

At the beginning of this book, I said that genetics and environment play an active role in our lives, but it seems that what we eat is vital to body organs and our well-being.

The best approach to improving immunity against autoimmune diseases, and inflammatory conditions or eating disorders, is to take a balanced, holistic multifaceted path towards health. Consider all the requirements necessary for your body, from various angles such as genetics, lifestyle and environment, eating healthy, to support or tackle the causes and not just the symptoms.

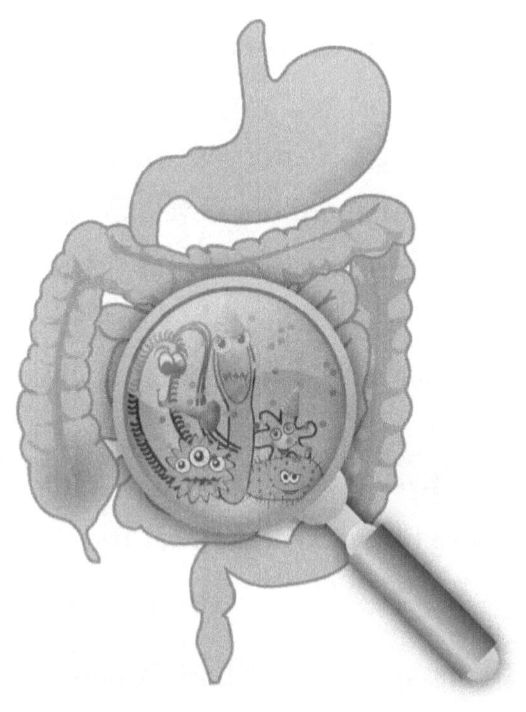

About the Author

Anthea Peries BSc (Hons) is a published author; she completed her undergraduate studies in several branches of the sciences, including Biology & Neurology, Brain and Behaviour and Child Development. A graduate member of the British Psychological Society, she has experience in counselling and is a former senior management executive. Born in London, Anthea enjoys fine, writing, and has travelled the world.

Thank you for reading this book. If you found it helpful, please recommend it to others, and if you have time, leave an honest review on Amazon.

You may also be interested in other
books by this author (see next page).

Other Books by This Author

- **Sugar Cravings:** How to Stop Sugar Addiction & Lose Weight.

- **Food Addiction**: Why You Eat to Fall Asleep and How to Overcome Night Eating Syndrome.

- **Food Addiction**: Overcoming Your Addiction to Sugar, Junk Food, and Binge Eating.

- **Food Addiction**: Overcome Sugar Bingeing, Overeating on Junk Food & Night Eating Syndrome.

- **Food Addiction:** Binge Eating Disorders.

- **Food Addiction**: Stop Binge Eating, Food Cravings and Night Eating, Overcome Your Addiction to Junk Food & Sugar.

- **Food Cravings**: Simple Strategies to Help Deal with Craving for Sugar & Junk Food.

- **Overcome Food Addiction**: How to Overcome Food Addiction, Binge Eating and Food Cravings.

- **Coping with Cancer:** *How Can You Help Someone with Cancer, Dealing with Cancer Family Member, Facing Cancer Alone, Dealing with Terminal Cancer Diagnosis, Chemotherapy Treatment & Recovery.*

- **Cancer: Chemotherapy Treatment Monitoring & Management**: *(Coping with Cancer, Oncology, Chemotherapy, After Side Effects), two manuscripts in 1.*

- **Chemotherapy:** *After Side Effects Chart, Cycle Journal & Medical Appointments Diary for Chemo, Oncology, Cancer Treatment & Recovery.*

- **Coping with Chemotherapy**: *After Side Effects and Recovery (Coping with Cancer, Cancer, Chemotherapy, After Side Effects)*
Two manuscripts in 1 or, a compendium of 2 books.

Fuck Cancer: *Chemotherapy Treatment Journal.*

For further information, please see
the Anthea's Amazon Author Page.